SPIRITUAL BALANCING

A Guidebook for Living in the Light

DIANA BURNEY

North Atlantic Books
Berkeley, California

Published by
North Atlantic Books
Berkeley, California

Cover photo © iStockphoto.com/AVTG
Cover design by Howie Severson
Interior design by Suzanne Albertson

Printed in the United States of America

Spiritual Balancing: A Guidebook for Living in the Light is sponsored and published by the Society for the Study of Native Arts and Sciences (dba North Atlantic Books), an educational nonprofit based in Berkeley, California, that collaborates with partners to develop cross-cultural perspectives, nurture holistic views of art, science, the humanities, and healing, and seed personal and global transformation by publishing work on the relationship of body, spirit, and nature.

North Atlantic Books' publications are available through most bookstores. For further information, visit our website at www.northatlanticbooks.com or call 800-733-3000.

Library of Congress Cataloging-in-Publication Data

Burney, Diana
    Spiritual balancing : a guidebook for living in the light / by Diana Burney.
        pages cm
    Summary: "A book about spiritual empowerment, Spiritual Balancing provides practical tools for clearing out negative energies, so that people can cease their struggles and accelerate their spiritual journey"—Provided by publisher.
    ISBN 978-1-58394-988-7 (trade)–ISBN 978-1-58394-989-4 (ebook)
    1. Spiritual life—Miscellanea. 2. Parapsychology. 3. Occultism. I. Title.
    BF1999.B7648 2016
    204'.4—dc23   2015013160
            1 2 3 4 5 6 7 8 9 UNITED 21 20 19 18 17 16

Printed on recycled paper

This book is dedicated to Avery and Quinn

CONTENTS

PREFACE

The information in this book is not new. Rather it contains ancient wisdom from various sources and spiritual teachers who have been instrumental in assisting me with navigating my spiritual journey over several decades. This book is a compendium of spiritually based practices that may be unfamiliar to a new seeker and, perhaps, forgotten by a seasoned one. My guidance was to research many spiritual practices that are not readily available so that individuals would have a variety of options to help them feel focused, safe, and secure as they fulfill their mission during this incarnation. In response to the considerable correspondence I received from my first book, I have revised the procedure for performing Spiritual Clearings for homes and properties so that those of different faiths can more easily implement it. Also, since God has many names in different religions and cultures, I have chosen to replace the word "God" with a universal description of "Source of All That Is." For the sake of brevity, I have reduced the phrase to the single word "Source." Then readers can insert whichever Divine name is comfortable for them.

Namasté

INTRODUCTION

(Automatic writing of July 1988)

My purpose in writing this book is to allow the reader to release blocks and doubts that spiritual enlightenment does not happen to "ordinary" individuals, but rather to those who are somehow blessed with a gift.

Nobody could have convinced me in my first few decades that what I have experienced on a spiritual level could have transpired. My life prior to my spiritual awakening in my thirties was simply going through the emotions. I have been touched and therefore I can touch others. It is with Universal Love that I share the essence of my rewarding spiritual climb, so that it might hasten or trigger you to commence with or complete your own inner work.

In this book I include exercises, techniques, and methods to ward off any negative energy attempting to dissuade you from your life's mission. Also included are practices to raise your vibratory rate as the Earth raises Hers.

It is my deepest desire that the reader will appreciate the material in this book and find it timeless in value. The information within can show how to embark on a higher path of life by employing the principles of intention, visualization, faith, and affirmation, all of which have important influences on health as well as spiritual development. Practicing the meditations, techniques, and exercises between the covers of this book can enhance spiritual perceptions.

By implementing the vibrational-shifting and life-transforming tools in this book, you can become spiritually empowered and thus connect to the higher Light and power of your heart and soul. May the Light of the Universe follow you throughout your spiritual journey.

Chapter 1

Moving Forward Spiritually

With the influx of higher-vibrational energies that have been flooding the planet since December 12, 2012, everyone on Earth has been affected in some manner. These energies are intermittently subtle and intense, influencing us all on multiple levels, some known and others unknown.

We are now living in a period where it is becoming increasingly acceptable for people to develop and embrace their spiritual side. More people than ever are awakening spiritually to opportunities that are outside the material world. As we awake, we raise our vibrations. As we raise our vibratory rate, we need to release the toxicity associated with our former way of being. Therefore, as the spiritual unfoldment continues, we will release any and all energies that cannot be sustained in a higher-vibrating reality. As a result, this process may allow us to become more sensitive to medications, herbs, essential oils, deodorants, lotions, aromas, homeopathic remedies, supplements, and foods.

This spiritual evolutionary process can occur at all levels of humanity including teachers, business people, farmers, politicians, and physicians. However, this process differs from one person to the next. No one can tell beforehand how long the individual spiritual-growth journey will take. For some the focus may be on physical symptoms, whereas for others the experience may be primarily emotional or psychological in nature. Many intense changes can occur both internally and externally that can be confusing or even bewildering.[1] The process will take as long as needed for each person.

What Is Spiritual Awakening?

A spiritual awakening occurs when a person becomes more aware of what is going on around and within him or her, on a much deeper and higher level. It is a life-changing shift in consciousness. A person will start to have a greater awareness of life experiences and begin to understand the reasons for these experiences and any lessons learned. The person will choose to let go of long-standing harbored emotions such as hurt, anger, resentment, and any other negative feelings or attitudes toward family of origin or others. This process occurs as the person gradually begins to heal heart, body, and soul. Every day is an opportunity to grow spiritually or to remain stagnant. The doorway for this experience is within each of us.

Every type of awakening is a remembering. It is the Light in us that is beginning to infiltrate our attention. We are beginning to remember other parts of ourselves that we had forgotten were even there. Spiritual awakening entails a potential radical departure in relation to our thoughts. The vibration of every thought impacts you. By shifting from a thought that is negative to one that is positive, you can raise your energy vibration and strengthen yourself and your immediate energy field. Your past becomes part of the Old, and the Old no longer matters. If things aren't going the way you would like them to go, just let go of that expectation. If something is not changing in your life, it is because you are choosing the same things over and over again. This new approach is about evaluating the foundation of your beliefs and being totally honest with your true situations and desires. We all have different abilities, characteristics, and strengths; however, every person has the ability to change instantaneously. Perhaps it is time now to choose or create something different.

Frequently people place blinders on to avoid the truth and deny the reality of their thoughts and feelings. One of the reasons people plug into denial is to (try to) avoid change. The New Earth requires that we act from the perspective of our Highest Good rather than from the external orientation of society. Please know that there is much Universal support for these changes. Mentors or teachers may appear everywhere with perfect timing to help you on your spiritual journey. Books may fall off shelves at your feet. Movies, events, teleseminars, and people who are meaningful will appear with synchronicity. In addition, spiritual guidance may arrive in your dreams. You are being called to fulfill your life purpose now. It is an awakening of your connection to Divine energy and is a doorway to develop mastery over your lower nature.

Being in the Now is the way of the New Earth. By "New Earth" I am referring to the changes taking place in our environment and in the consciousness of many of us. New, unexplained, and previously unknown energies have entered the planet, and your body is not familiar with them and has no frame of reference for coping or interacting. As these higher frequencies of Light rapidly intensify, they are creating alchemical changes within our existing structures. This process is quickly changing the fundamental foundations of our planet, human bodies, psyches, consciousness, and DNA. This infusion of Light is stressful and is creating a large-scale purification process, which is affecting everything and everybody on Earth, according to the sensitivity of each person.

Everything is changing as we all move together into a new state of being and let go of third-dimensional concepts. We will be unable to take these old values and ways of existing into the infrastructure of the New Earth and its Unity Consciousness. If we were already operating at the higher energetic levels, then we wouldn't have to deal with the issues of fear, anger, depression, and pain that are present worldwide right now. As we move into a higher vibration, our energies are no longer in alignment with these lower-density emotions.

As people begin their individual process toward a full awakening consciousness, they start to face their fears, release emotional blocks, and clear away negativity in as many areas of life as possible. This involves releasing painful trapped negative emotions of the past. Often, the process of awakening spiritually can be very confusing and so powerful that people may begin to question their sanity. I remember vividly an experience I had once when I was washing my hair in my pedestal sink at home in my bathroom. After the final rinse, I lifted my head from the sink and found myself totally disoriented as to where I was. I looked in my mirror but did not recognize what I was viewing. This experience lasted for seconds only, but it was very unsettling, to say the least. It took me several weeks to understand the significance of that event, and that my altered state of perception was due to a shift in vibration.

Increasing awareness of synchronicities and life lessons results in viewing the world from a different perspective and re-evaluating one's previous opinions, judgments, and beliefs. You may realize that there is more to life than you have been taught to believe. Since spiritual awakening is a personal journey, it differs from one individual to another, in type of episodes as well as duration. For some, it may occur spontaneously from a near-death experience or a profound emotional and/or spiritual incident. For others, it can be a gradual process with messages in dreams, classes taken, a Kundalini experience, bodywork, or anything that sparks the activation of awareness. This spiritual awakening process may take days or even years and is dependent on how long a person chooses to hold on to fear, anger, sadness, and other lower-vibrational emotions. It is an evolutionary process of seeking spiritual growth and development, and it happens differently for everyone. Following are fifty of the more common signs and symptoms of a spiritual awakening process, but it is not a conclusive list by any means.

Some of the symptoms listed below are being experienced by many people. However, these symptoms are all temporary. They indicate that physiological changes to assist the physical body in its journey into higher-vibrational frequencies are occurring so we can exist on higher dimensional levels as our vibrations increase.[2]

Taking care of the physical body becomes more important now.

Once the spiritual awakening process is completed, an individual will be more heart-centered and have more empathy and compassion for others. At the same time, he or she will continue to learn new lessons and acquire additional knowledge with a new and different perspective and a heightened awareness.

Spiritual Awakening Symptoms

- Inconsistent sleep patterns such as restlessness or frequent waking
- Sudden waves of emotion, especially anger, fear, and sadness
- Headaches, backaches, pains in neck and shoulders
- Feelings of being different than you were previously
- Vivid or intense dreams
- Dizzy spells and feeling lightheaded
- Tingling in your crown and third-eye chakras or hands and feet
- New food and drink intolerances and allergies
- Feeling more tired and needing to rest more than usual
- A desire for freedom from stressful jobs and toxic people
- Feeling like you have a brain fog
- Energy surges moving through your body
- Emotional confusion
- A sense that time is speeding up
- Memory loss and forgetfulness
- Unusual food cravings
- An increase in synchronicity and coincidences
- A feeling of losing your mind
- Senses become more enhanced and may become overloaded
- An increase in creative bursts of inspiration
- Disinterest in sex
- Intense mood swings
- Wanting to withdraw from family or friends
- Searching for your purpose
- Occurrence of a life-altering event
- An interest in spirituality for the first time
- Unusual physical maladies such as nausea and numbness

- A change in what you choose to read or do
- Heart palpitations or feeling that your heart is racing
- Increased intuition
- Feeling as though your life is out of control
- Spiritual teachers or advisors suddenly appear
- Sudden awareness of recurring patterns
- Apathy or loss of motivation
- May become aware of psychic gifts or healing abilities
- Seeing the message in everything that occurs
- Increased sensitivity or empathy toward others
- May choose to take better care of your physical body
- An intense desire for a spiritual partner
- Desire to break old habits and start new routines
- Increased integrity
- Bouts of depression for no real reason
- Ringing in the ears
- Attunement with nature
- Desire to discover spiritual truths
- Sense of inner peace
- Feeling ungrounded
- Increased ability to manifest
- Sensing other dimensions
- Yearning for a simpler lifestyle

Easing Spiritual Awakening

First of all, check with your physician to make sure that none of the symptoms you are experiencing are due to a medical condition. Once you are medically cleared, the following suggestions may help you restore equilibrium. If your symptoms are not intense, the best way to cope is to become grounded and to meditate.

- Take the time to be out in nature daily, whether it be taking a walk or sitting in a park or garden setting. Being close to a water source can be very soothing.
- Read articles, blogs, and books on spiritual awakening.
- Confide to a trusted friend what you are experiencing, for moral support.
- Incorporate mindfulness, chanting, praying, or singing with daily activities such as walking, yoga, dancing, eating, or meditation.
- Receive bodywork whenever possible, such as cranial-sacral and other massage, acupuncture, chiropractic, Reiki, or other energetic healing modalities.
- Take one- or two-minute abdominal breathing breaks throughout the day.
- Drink plenty of water.
- Learn to ask for help when you need it.
- Move your body through stretching, yoga, or dance to release any energy blockages.
- Pay close attention to your thoughts, words, and actions.
- Seek out the guidance of a spiritual group or circle.
- Use Bach Flower Essences and the other Spiritual Power Tools in this book.
- Play inspirational music or an instrument, and create a spiritual playlist.
- Interact more with the animal kingdom.
- Be loving to yourself for having the courage to release outmoded patterns.
- Begin a daily journal of your meditations, revelations, and experiences.
- Routinely balance your chakras and clear your aura.
- Maintain daily spiritual protection and don't leave home without it!

- Get out of your own way and let go of what no longer serves you.

- Reevaluate your eating choices and avoid lower-vibrational foods such as processed foods, GMO (soy, corn, wheat), and especially refined sugar.

- Ask your Higher Self to guide you to a spiritual teacher.

- Locate a trusted healthcare professional who can work with your inner guidance.

- To the mind, surrendering to Source can feel like death, so be prepared for fear to arise. If it does, you can then tap it away with the Emotional Freedom Technique. By voicing positive affirmations while gently tapping your fingertips on specific energy meridians, the balance of mind and body can be restored.

Be aware that the mind creates your reality. Consequently, if it feels that it could be ignored, then it can create unusual experiences to distract you from achieving your goal of spiritual awakening.[3] Old patterns and behaviors are being pushed to the surface for release.

Since your vibrations are shifting as well as your emotions, it is best to have a variety of spiritual options available to you. There are many described in this book that can be effective to gain balance in your environment for different situations. For example, if meditation isn't helpful, then try prayer or chanting. If that doesn't seem to be effective, then schedule a bodywork or counseling session. Everyone processes issues at a different pace.

Just remember: you are changing for the better; you are heading for a life of deeper fulfillment and purpose. As you do, you will find different ways to pass the time and may not enjoy activities you have always pursued as much anymore. You'll find new pastimes that will interest you. Just be open to what comes your way, and surround yourself with people who are positive and inspire you.

Change and growth are taking place; the discomfort you experience is increased by resistance. Know that all is exactly as it should be, and you are having the human experience of growth. When discomfort strikes, ask yourself where or what you are resisting and then let it go. Between living up to work demands and family expectations, sometimes you can feel a bit overwhelmed ... then your spiritual acceleration overlays all that.

My Changes

When I first embarked on my spiritual journey in 1983, there was very little information available to educate and prepare me for the plethora of experiences that I encountered. In fact, it might be difficult to believe, but even books on astrology were often hidden in the back of large chain bookstores under the heading of "Occult." Infrequently, if I searched in the "Religion" section of these same commercial bookstores, I would find some "mystical" or metaphysical morsels of information that I could apply to what was occurring in my life. However, the vast majority of my understanding and knowledge was gained through my twice-weekly sessions with my Eastern Indian meditation teacher, Raj. He referred me to several older esoteric books written by Charles W. Leadbeater, which were interesting but difficult to read. Then he referred me to *Autobiography of a Yogi* by Paramahansa Yogananda, and it inspired me to search even further for information about developing spiritually.

This search guided me first in the direction of Spiritualism, a movement based on the belief that those who have passed over can communicate with those who are still living. Ultimately, I became an ordained Spiritualist Minister while living in Sedona, Arizona, in 1993. The following year, I became a Reiki Master/Teacher, which then led me down my path as a Healer and on to becoming a present-day Spiritual Teacher and an author.

Since spiritual growth is an "inside job," and everyone has different body chemistry, temperaments, and experiences, I will not bore you with all the details of my journey. While the listing of all my physical, mental, emotional, and spiritual adjustments had my family labeling me a hypochondriac, those personal details are beyond the scope of this book. However, I am guided to share some of the "solutions" that I found to be the most helpful. Please realize that this is a reference list of what I found to be of great assistance to me. I do not have any agreement or partnership with any of the companies or products listed. These recommendations are only informational in the event that you are also struggling with some of the issues I have resolved using the products named. It is also important for you to know that the discovery of these solutions for me took many years of trial and error, and dollars wasted with other possibilities. Also, know that some of these products are more costly than expected and were purchased one at a time over many months as I could allocate the expenses in my budget. So please don't think you have to purchase everything at once. It would be best if you prioritized what would be the most beneficial for the symptoms you are experiencing. These symptoms are not listed chronologically or in any particular order other than how they showed up in my mind as I was writing about this topic.

- I am unable to wear synthetic fabrics because they make my skin itchy, so I read all fabric labels and stick to three types: cotton, silk, and rayon. Furthermore, I prefer bright-colored clothing and have difficulty wearing anything that is black.

- This fabric issue extends to my choice of bedding. Many popular manmade fabrics used to create sheets, comforters, and pillowcases contain harsh, dangerous chemicals. After many years of searching, I discovered that I sleep more soundly when I use cotton sheets that have a high thread count. My mattress is extremely important, and I have found that I sleep better on a 100% natural latex mattress on a heavy-duty wood foundation.

- Long ago, I developed lactose intolerance before it became a consumer issue. Instead, I drink organic almond, rice, or coconut milk.

- I have developed a considerable number of food allergies, especially to garlic and spicy foods. Dye-Free Benadryl and GOLD (not regular) Alka Seltzer are helpful if I can't avoid those types of food.

- Artificial flavorings make me nauseous, so I add essential oils or organic extracts if I want flavorings. Over the years, I have simply chosen to eat foods plain. At the dentist, I prefer plain dental cleaning paste over artificial flavor choices. I am unable to use an electric toothbrush, as it sends tiny electrical shocks through my teeth.

- Speaking of dental-related issues, I have developed multiple sensitivities to many dental products. Consequently, every several years I obtain blood work to determine which dental products are compatible with my physiology. These kits can be obtained from Clifford Consulting and Research Laboratory at www .ccrlab.com. The cost may seem high, but since I have had a considerable amount of dental issues, I'd rather be healthy.

- Regarding personal care products, I have had success with primarily using unscented organic deodorants, suntan lotion, hair products, cosmetics, and skin creams.

- For me, everything I use has to be unscented and non-toxic including candles, tissues (without lotions), laundry detergents, dryer sheets, etc. However, I do utilize organic essential oils for many household and personal uses.

- I am also extremely sensitive to the harmful energies of electromagnetic fields (EMFs) that are associated with electrical appliances such as televisions, computers, microwaves, cell phones (and land-lines), Smart Meters, breaker boxes, electrical transformers, cell phone towers, and Wi-Fi. So how do I function, you might ask. Ten years ago, I gave away my microwave oven, and I have never missed it. I depend on various gifts of the mineral kingdom and have grounding stones placed near or on electrical outlets. I do not have Wi-Fi capabilities in my home, and my high-speed internet runs through underground cables.

- Besides wearing natural grounding stones for years, I was fortunate to locate a company called Earth Calm (www.earthcalm .com) that makes technology devices for EMF protection. I constantly wear a sterling silver Nova Resonator Pendant, and I have purchased the Home EMF Protection System for myself and my family. When I travel, I plug in a Stetzerizer filter (www .stetzerizer-us.com) in the room where I sleep.

- I would like to share a technology that I have just become acquainted with in the past four years. It is the principle of Earthing, and the company is found online at www.Earthing .com. They have a huge selection of Earthing (grounding) products and starter kits. I have purchased all of the types of bed sheets, mats, travel sheets, and other products, and they have improved my physical health on so many levels. If you want more information, you can purchase the book by the same name.

- Additionally, I developed chlorine sensitivity. This condition was remedied by the purchase of a bath ball filter and a shower filter.

- My goal is to drink two liters of water daily, often with liquid minerals added.

- When taking any over-the-counter medication, I routinely start with the pediatric dosage and then increase the dose as I can tolerate.

- For the perpetual grayness of the winter months, I have sat in front of a broad-spectrum light every morning for decades.

- For improved sleep, I rely on an air purifier in my bedroom, and I also use a humidifier in the winter. My furnace filters must be changed at least monthly.

Traveling Precautions

When traveling, I am particularly challenged to reduce my exposure to electromagnetic frequencies (EMFs). Consequently, I employ a number of strategies to maintain the integrity of my energy field. Before entering an airport (or anywhere with large crowds), I consciously pull in my energetic fields. Through focus and intention, I ask the Universe to condense my auric bodies all into my physical body so that I don't absorb unwanted energies from others.

This technique has been extremely beneficial in preventing me from absorbing negative thought-forms and energies when walking through public places. However, it only lasts for a few hours and then my aura automatically returns to my normal energy field.

The following strategies are what I routinely and automatically do, in no particular order, when I arrive at my destination when traveling:

- Remove electrical appliances near my pillow, especially electric alarm clocks.

- Spray the bottom bed sheet, pillow, and tub and shower with sage aromatherapy spray.

- Ask Master St. Germain to blaze the Violet Transmuting Flame within, around, and through my room and bed.

- Cover the TV screen with a towel, or unplug it altogether, to reduce EMF radiation (even when the TV is not on).

- Plug in my Stetzerizer filter (www.stetzerizer-us.com).

- Set up a portable altar with a few favorite spiritual pictures and artifacts.

- Decline room service each day at the front desk and keep the privacy sign on the door to reduce outside discordant energies.

- Apply my Earthing half sheet (www.earthing.com) to my bed.

- Put my silk pillowcase on a pillow to protect me from scratchy pillowcases (www.naturalorganicway.com/product /DreamSacks-Silk-Pillowcase).

- Add my battery-operated travel alarm clock to the nightstand.

- Ask the Universe to place a Blue Cross etherically in the middle of my room and on all my doors and windows.

- Surround my room with the blue bubble of Divine power, the gold bubble of Divine wisdom, and the pink bubble of Divine love.

This little "nesting" procedure of mine probably sounds daunting to you, but I assure you that everything that I listed takes only a few minutes to implement.

The Energy of Thoughts

Thoughts are vibrating creative forces, and all actions are the result of thoughts. Nothing evolves without thought. If we think positively then that positive attitude will be reflected back to us through positive life experiences. Thoughts are created by desires or emotions. Desires or emotions are the survival outcomes of one or the other of the four basic human instincts: self-preservation, food, sex, and sleep. By controlling desires and emotions, thoughts can also be controlled. Thoughts are not passive images. They are powerful, vibrant energy patterns that eventually have to translate into action. Pay attention to how your thoughts emerge randomly and then begin to connect to other thoughts. You will eventually develop awareness that you are not your thoughts.

Through the practice of meditation, we can learn how to control our thoughts effectively. When thoughts are in control, actions resulting from those thoughts are also in control. You are here on Earth to develop mastery. By developing the skill of not reacting when challenged emotionally, you are in essence becoming a Master of your emotions. As you focus on those situations where you lose your emotional or mental balance, you can begin to identify further opportunities to grow spiritually.

As discussed by Jasmuheen in her book *In Resonance*, we are taught our thinking processes from those who teach us in our childhood years. Some of these processes have caused us to over-generalize; to think only in terms of black and white; to draw conclusions without evidence; to take everything personally; to always focus on our failures or our problems; to assume the worst in a situation; and to blow things out of proportion.[4]

Since these tendencies and situations have developed us into the people we are today, it is important that we avoid focusing on blame when reviewing our upbringing. The main reason it might be helpful to try to develop knowledge of the way we were raised is to better understand why certain behavior exists. In order to free ourselves from these limited patterns of thinking, we must become aware that thoughts are energy and can trigger emotions: we have the power to create our personal reality. Awareness creates choice, and choice often creates change. Change, then, happens when you are willing to take responsibility for both your strengths and limitations and seek to become a better, healthier, and more compassionate individual.

The vibrations of thought are ever present. You attract the current for which you are in harmony. Thought and image seek their own. The more pure, sincere, and constructive your thoughts, the higher will be the rate of your vibration. Just as the Light radiates, so must you, for you are a human radiator. It should be the aim of every individual to increase his or her radiation by positive thought, to rise to a higher vibration of love, harmony, and compassion.[5] The general characteristics of your thought world form the background for your aura. Thoughts of hope, inspiration, joy, anger, fear, optimism, peace, and love all radiate at a different vibration and color.[6]

Whatever manifests in your outer world is created first in your inner world. The energy that follows thought, and that you are constantly experiencing in your life, is the result of whatever resonates with the vibration you set in motion with your thoughts. The world around you is mirroring the world within you via your subconscious mind. Physical pains are often the outcome of some mental state you are experiencing on a subconscious level. It is best to throw out any thought that is negative and to cease to worry about "things." Should any negative thought enter your mind, do not dwell upon it or worry about it. Instead, just let it pass by without it affecting you. Keep tuning into the higher vibration. In the words of Dr. Murdo MacDonald-Bayne: "Speak from your heart, feel from your heart, and your head will follow suit."[7] Like attracts like; positivity attracts positivity; forgiveness attracts forgiveness; and happiness attracts happiness.[8]

Every atom in the Universe is vibrating at a specific frequency, and it is that frequency that you translate into the visible and invisible experiences through your senses. While you are in a physical body, you vibrate at a lower frequency than when you shed your physical unit, which is quite dense. Many people can sense the higher frequencies of angels or other energies, and a few individuals can "see" them with their inner vision.

Many people claim that they are unable to keep from thinking about a particular subject or situation. However, habits can change. You must choose not to give power to any aspect of your Being that is providing false information. This can take the form of prejudices, cultural biases, narrow-mindedness, or religious beliefs. The mental body is the perfect example of where misinformation is stored. Over the years of your lifetime, you have created many erroneous thoughts based on pure illusions. They seem totally real and have even provided a reference for judgments of yourself and others. What would it take to allow yourself to remain open to new ideas and question old beliefs? Your senses are not always reliable, as they do not provide you with the total picture of any given situation. Once emotional triggers are released, you will no longer magnetize negative situations to you. Rather than condemning yourself when you lose composure, take it in stride. Be grateful for the opportunity to reveal still another chance to heal an unresolved issue. This then will become a strength instead of a liability.

Personal power is lost when a person falls into the trap of reacting. Once it becomes apparent to you, you will stop falling for the situation. When you begin to see your reactions and analyze them properly, then you will see where your thoughts are focused. From the time you get up in the morning until you go to bed at night, your thoughts, emotions, and daily reactions have an effect upon your mind and physical body. Conditions exist internally long before they appear externally. These are invisible when they are in the mental or emotional state, but when they are transferred to the physical body they become a manifestation of those states.[9]

Changing your responses is also an "inside job," and the quicker you decide to embrace the opportunity, the happier you will become. It doesn't matter when you decide to make a change, because the present moment is all that is important. Welcome change as you would a new friend and learn to stay in the moment, as that is all there is. The past is over, and the future has not yet arrived.

As I stated previously, awareness is the starting point for all change to occur. It is at this point that you can begin to optimize the plan for your life as you realize your progress or lack of progress in certain areas. Reaching this point can be accelerated by establishing goals from that place of inner power. Then synchronize the goals with the energy of intention for their realization.

You are provided with every conceivable opportunity to accomplish exactly what you came to this planet to achieve, and you must open your mind to these opportunities. Verbalizing this is far easier than implementing it for most of us. Although you must initiate the process to have a chance to reach your spiritual destination, sometimes it is very important to demonstrate a physical move toward a goal to release the stagnation.

At times it is overwhelming to individuals to think about change even when they are fully cognizant that their lives are not fulfilling their needs, and they are not accomplishing their goals. At the time when this realization is made, there are two main options available to you. You can override the realization and continue doing what you are doing. This choice will allow you more opportunities to feel uncomfortable with your current path and provide you with a chance to make another life change later. The other option is to make a decision to take a more productive path through this choice and become more serious and committed about your responsibilities. When you choose to change, you can accelerate the success of the changes through your prayers and meditation. By requesting assistance from your heart, you will often be given all the guidance that is appropriate for your intentions.

Free will exists in every moment. Each individual makes his or her choice about every aspect of life. Now is the time to reprogram your conscious mind. What is causing your suffering is not the circumstances you are in, but rather your thoughts about those circumstances. You are creating a story in your mind about the situation. You choose your reality. You are in charge of how you feel. When you realize this fact, then you have control. Become aware of your thoughts and what you are telling yourself. By shifting from a thought that is negative to one that is positive, you can raise your energy vibration and strengthen yourself and alter your immediate energy field. Next, reprogram your subconscious mind and increase your vibrations.

The choice of what vibration you want to attract in your life is yours in every moment. You can choose to release the energy of a positive thought-form or a negative one. All is energy, and all energy follows thought. You create what you think. Words become things. A positive attitude can uplift the people around you as well as raise your own vibratory rate. Consequently, with everything you say, think, do, and feel, you are always either contributing to the Light or adding to the darkness of this planet. You are a product of thought. All thoughts—your own, those of others, and the collective world thought—affect us.

All thoughts summon a response from the Universe. All your thoughts will either contribute to your healing, and therefore the world's healing, or they will postpone healing. When you focus your thinking on what you want to avoid, or what is fearful or painful to you or another, you are giving energy and focus to what you *don't* want to occur. When your life doesn't appear to be positive, stop and ask yourself: *"Why am I telling myself this now?"* and follow up with: *"Why am I giving myself this experience?"* Since a belief is what you consider to be true, to know what you truly believe, simply watch what you do. You may talk differently, but you always do what you believe. Your behavior will tell the truth about who you really are.

Paying attention is key. The simple task of observing and acknowledging which thoughts, words, emotions, and actions you are choosing is very important. The stresses and challenges of your life condition often accumulate beneath your awareness. This process results in a plethora of emotional responses and often creates physical maladies. We easily get caught up in the human condition and lose sight of opportunities to find peace and balance. Sometimes we are so overwhelmed by our thoughts and worries that we simply shut down, as it is the only method we know to regain a sense of equilibrium. We feel out of sync. We forget that we created our own gerbil-wheel existence and that we can choose to take ourselves off the gerbil wheel and restore harmony in our lives.

Most of us live in a quasi-trance and are running on automatic pilot. In your overstressed life, you may be barely able to remember what you did yesterday, much less be aware as you are doing it. That is the problem. Until you are paying attention, you cannot measure your spiritual progress. As a result, you cannot know accurately where you are on your journey to spiritual growth and may overestimate your spiritual expertise.

As you become more aware of your thoughts, you realize how much time you have wasted with stagnant thinking. Much energy has been expended thinking about the past, the future, or judgments. Your thoughts originate from your childhood beliefs, your religious affiliations, your attitudes, your values, your education, your peers, and what you see, read, and hear in the media. Did you know that thoughts and emotions can be absorbed from others and then accepted as your own? Like attracts like, so in time, similar thought energies begin to be embraced by an individual, affecting every thought and action. Most people believe that thoughts are involuntary and that they cannot help thinking what they think. This is an erroneous assumption, because even the most obsessive thinking can be restrained and reframed.

As a result, it is vital that you listen to what you say to others, watch your actions, and notice your thoughts. By observing your thoughts, interactions, and behaviors you will soon be able to discern what people and situations are triggers for negative thinking, and which unwanted emotions are the most frequent for you to adjust to and overcome. This revelation is truly present-moment living. Change your habits through your thoughts, feelings, words, and actions. That which you think and do and feel qualifies your energy, and that energy is what you emit into your emotional body.[10]

Your moods connect you vibrationally with other similar moods. The best that you can do to avoid acting as a channel for the mass consciousness is simply to be self-aware. This situation is easier said than done when you are overwhelmed by your feelings, but simply knowing about this energy reality is the beginning of self-awareness and wise self-control. It is a good idea to monitor yourself after extreme moods and access how much of the emotional charge was actually yours, and then commit yourself to a lower volume next time. Simply understanding these realities may be enough to help you change.

You will also understand the importance of your personal behavior. Your moods and thoughts do not simply affect you and those closest to you. They affect everyone. At the same time, your self-control and transformation can benefit others as well, for negative thinking is very similar to negative speaking. The primary difference is that the spoken word takes shape in the physical/auditory realm, while the thought remains in the etheric/astral/mental realm. Both words and thoughts infiltrate the auras of both the speaker/thinker and the one to whom that thought or word is directed. Consequently, through the law of attraction, they both call forth whatever is the focus of the manifestation.[11]

The human body is an electrified body, sending out vibrations or radiations. The outside radiations influence us according to what we are attracting. We attract the same conditions that we radiate. We radiate the vibrations of our dominant thoughts and emotions.[12] One way to change this situation is to invoke your I AM Presence to regulate your thoughts and then visualize the Light from within those little electrons blazing out through those thoughts and causing them to increase the vibration of their motion around their central core.[13]

The I AM Presence

The I AM Presence is the spiritual body that is the highest in vibration and extends beyond the other energy bodies. It is the purest part of you and is the spark of Divinity. As you merge with your I AM, you once again become Oneness. It is your Divine intelligence.[14] The I AM Presence is an Immortal Body of Light Substance that connects the Divinity in every human being with Source, which is the reality of your True Self. It is from this "Divine Ray of Light" that you receive your Light, life, intelligence, energy, and physical being. There is an invisible stream of electronic Light that runs from your I AM Presence down through your crown chakra to anchor in your physical heart that is known as the "Silver Cord." This Divine Ray of Light unites each individualized I AM Presence with Source.[15]

The words "I AM" are the creative words of the Universe. Thus, when using these creative words you should always follow with a positive and constructive statement, as your I AM Presence is Source within you. In this manner, your subconscious mind will accept and imprint within itself every statement that follows these creative words.[16] "I AM" pays direct acknowledgment to the Source/God within.[17] Examples would be: *"I AM one with all there is"* and *"I AM choosing only positive thoughts now."* Saying an affirmation is like making a statement, so it is important that you say it with as much conviction and emotion as possible. When you utilize affirmations, it is imperative that you release ALL attachments to the results once you make the statements. When you attach yourself to the results of wanting or being something, you actually can have the opposite effect occur and then repel the condition away from you.

Life on the New Earth

The configuration of the Earth's magnetic field is changing. Like it or not, we are moving with rapid speed toward a new and as yet undefined world. The new higher frequencies streaming to the Earth are bringing in new opportunities with a new paradigm. This new paradigm is about being happy and finding your joy. It's about aligning your life with your soul's mission and purpose. It's about making the right choices each and every day and choosing acceptance, verbalizing gratitude, exercising compassion, and "paying it forward" by helping others for no other reason except that you can. These choices are based on your intuition and not on someone's expectation of your life. The only way you can truly be happy is to release judgments about yourself and others and initiate the necessary steps to take charge of your life. Each of us has the power to participate in actually molding and recreating a better world. This mission can be accomplished by becoming responsible for our individual actions and choices. For it is the sum total of each of our actions and choices that will move the world in any given direction.

Life on this New Earth is about becoming serious about your life, taking responsibility for your spiritual development, and fulfilling your life's purpose. Each person has a unique purpose in every lifetime. By placing your attention on understanding your life's purpose, you will receive information and guidance about it. Melding with this new paradigm is easier to read about than actually to implement the changes and then to sustain them. It is much easier to decide on making a change than to ultimately make it permanent. It is counterproductive to start too many changes and not follow through with them. Past lack of success with reaching goals may create future resistance. However, by acknowledging that your life was orchestrated in order for you to fulfill your destiny, you can release your victim and poverty consciousness and move forward one courageous step at a time. These small steps can set in motion a major directional shift in your life.

The most important part to remember is that each day is a brand new opportunity to make changes and to make choices in your life. Then begin to realize that your life begins as a clear slate each minute in every day. In each and every moment, you have a choice to contribute in a positive or negative way to your life. It is time to embrace this new crossroad and become aware of the new choices that were not available to you in the past. Awareness is the key. By identifying patterns in your relationships and situations, you can accelerate the release and finally break the cycle. Observe all that you are experiencing rather than be concerned about the future and what may never even happen. There is no past, and there is no future, only the present moment. Everyone has written his or her own play at this time for a reason, and the reason is to learn lessons. When you lose your focus on the moment by distracting yourself with concerns about the future or what is lacking, you also lose your focus on your life's lessons.

The New Earth is about weaving new concepts into the tapestry of your life, and about being patient. It is about trusting the process and having faith that positive changes are occurring for your Highest Good. These changes are happening even if you do not have any direct acknowledgment of them.

Another obstacle to the new paradigm is your erroneous beliefs and misconceptions. Through your awareness of any self-imposed obstacles, and other self-sabotaging behaviors, you take a major step forward to overcome that limitation. That is half the battle. The other half is a combination of being motivated to change and discovering an appropriate method to accomplish that. There is always time to change, and this very moment is a perfect time to commit or reaffirm your intention to be open to a transformation.

Time and space are illusions we create for ourselves in the third-dimensional reality. In the Universe, however, there is no time or space.

On Earth, we apparently need the concept of time and space to assist us to organize our thoughts and tasks into a linear frame of reference to make it easier to sort through our experiences. As we move into higher frequencies and expand our consciousness, the acceleration process frees our Being to access information at remarkable speeds. This acceleration of information occurs when we move beyond the density of the third-dimensional reality. We accomplish this movement into the higher realms through intention, daily practices, breathing exercises, focus, meditation, and prayers. Breathing exercises especially will increase the life-force energy within your body. If you are interested in increasing your storehouse of energy, you would be wise to dedicate time each day to some of the wonderful breathing techniques listed throughout this book, in order to increase your life-force reserves.

Now more than ever, you have the opportunity to make a difference for the planet and all of humanity as a whole. Choosing to pursue another direction will require a serious commitment. Being successful will depend on your unwavering focus on the goal you set and breaking the many habits that have formed around the role you are leaving behind. Embrace the changes in every phase of your life and allow your True Self to unfold more fully every day in every way.

Your intentions determine the support received, and this is a very important point to consider. You may seek assistance with one aspect of your life and receive the necessary help with that aspect. You may also take a broad view of your life and consider your requests from the vantage point of a "higher mind," therefore gaining a much greater perspective and discovering a deeper understanding.

Throughout your lifetime, you have had the opportunity to experience the surge of a variety of strong emotions. Unfortunately, many times there was no outlet for them. Other times it was inappropriate to unleash the full intensity of the emotions that were felt. Consequently, these emotions were squelched, banished, and stored. Sometimes they were forgotten and buried in the recesses of your mind and body. Assuming that these intense, energetic waves of emotions have disappeared, you continue through your life sojourn unaware of their dormant existence.

Emotions have energy and intensity of their own that eventually rise to the surface, often at awkward times. This naturally creates confusion and vulnerability when it occurs. The people expressing the feelings are bewildered because they thought they had already dealt with the events and root causes at an earlier point in time. Those witnessing the verbal release are often caught off guard. Thoughts are things. Every thought creates a set of correlated vibrations in the matter of the mental body. The mental body under this impulse throws off a vibrating portion of itself, created by the nature of the vibrations. This gathers from the surrounding atmosphere energy like itself in fineness from the elemental essence of the mental world. We have then a thought-form pure and simple. And it is a living entity of intense activity animated by the one idea that generated it.[18]

Similar to other vibrations, these thought-forms tend to reproduce themselves whenever an opportunity is offered to them, and so when they strike upon another mental body they tend to provoke it at their own rate and motion. In other words, they tend to produce in the mind of others thoughts of the same type as that which was sent forth in waves from the thinker. From the point of view of the individual whose mental body is touched by these waves—they tend to produce in their mind thoughts of the same type as that which had previously arisen in the mind of the thinker who sent forth the waves. The distance to which such thought-waves penetrate, and the force and persistence with which they impinge upon the mental bodies of others, depend on the strength and clarity of the original thought.[19]

Each person moves through life enclosed within a case of their building, surrounded by a mass of the forms created by their own habitual thoughts. Through this medium, a person views the world, and naturally he or she sees everything tinged with its predominant colors and all rates of vibration similar to their own. Consequently, until humans learn complete control of their thoughts and feelings, they see nothing as it really is, since all their observations are viewed through this medium, which distorts and colors everything like poorly made glass.

If a thought-form is not personal or directly aimed at someone else, it simply floats detached in the atmosphere, all the time radiating vibrations similar to those originally set forth by its creator. If it does not come in contact with any other mental body, the vibration gradually exhausts its store of energy and, in that case, disintegrates. However, if it succeeds in awakening a similar vibration in any mental body nearby, an attraction is formed, and that mental body usually absorbs the thought-form.[20]

Thought-forms directed toward individuals produce marked effects. These effects are either partially reproduced in the aura of the receiver, increasing the total result, or repelled from it. Any combination of energy can only vibrate within certain definite limits, and if the thought-form is outside the limits within which the aura is capable of vibrating, it cannot affect that aura at all. It consequently rebounds from it with a force proportionate to the energy that it impinged upon the aura.[21]

The key is for you to be aware that every single situation that you have ever experienced is stored as an emotional imprint somewhere within your body structure. For instance, if you had difficulty expressing anger constructively as you were growing up, there will be layers of anger stored within your body. Each layer is the result of each separate event where anger was not expressed in a healthy manner. Frequently, this type of experience will result in some level of depression and negativity that will follow you throughout your lifetime. The same occurs for all other emotions such as anxiety, fear, shame, grief, worry, and guilt. Besides the physical body, these emotions can be stored in your chakras and your aura.

Every thought, word, emotion, and action is a vibration that creates your aura. The aura is a beautiful three-dimensional field of ever-changing energy patterns that surrounds your physical body in all directions. The healthier you are, physically and spiritually, the more vibrant your aura will be. Your aura is a physical manifestation of your soul. However, this human aura is generally not stable and changes according to both internal and external stimuli.[22]

This human aura is created by the thoughts and feelings, both conscious and subconscious, that are taking place within you. Wherever your thoughts are focused, so are your auric energy patterns. Just as an electromagnetic field is caused by the electric current flowing through its wire, the auric field is caused by the thoughts and feelings that are flowing within your conscious and subconscious minds and the interplay between the two. As your thoughts and feelings change, so do the colors that are emanated into your auric field. Learning to perceive and control your aura helps you become more aware of energy patterns of thought that you project and have projected at you throughout the day. The more sensitive you become to your aura, the more you can recognize and control what energies you allow into and out of it.[23]

Each person's energy field is unique unto itself. No two energy fields are entirely alike. There may be similarities, but each person has a signature frequency. Most people can feel the auras of those around them. Have you noticed that when you are physically close to someone who is angry and upset you feel uneasy and want to move away from them, or that when you are with someone who is relaxed and happy you enjoy staying close to them? Have you ever been able to sense how someone is feeling, in spite of how that person acted? When you are around some people, do you feel drained? Have you ever felt when someone was staring at you? If you answered "yes" to any of these questions, you have experienced the interplay of an outside energy field upon your aura.[24]

Due to the strong electromagnetic properties of the aura, you constantly release and absorb energy. Each time you come in contact with someone, an exchange of energy can occur. The more people you interact with, the greater the energy exchanges. That is why it is so important to understand how your aura is affected by others and how your aura affects them. Keeping your frequency elevated with positive and uplifting thoughts can affect your family and all others in a harmonious way.

To make the most of life on the New Earth, you must be aware of the Universal Life Force flowing through you in every moment. By remaining in the present moment, you create a synergy with this Divine energy. When you become distracted by trivial concerns about the past or the future that you have no control over, you miss the golden opportunities that are placed before you each day.

Chapter 2

Coping with the Ascension Process

The word "ascension" generally refers to a physically upward motion through space. However, in the context of human spiritual evolution, this term describes the acceleration of the vibratory action of the atoms of the physical body through spiritual practices and exercises.[1] Ascension in this sense is not so much a mystical experience as it is a scientific one. The electrons that compose the atoms of an individual's inner and physical auric bodies vibrate at the speed of the consciousness of that individual. The slower the vibrations, the more connection an individual has with like vibrations of the lower densities on Earth. At the same time, the awakening consciousness of individuals who desire to fulfill their Divine Plan will quicken their vibrations. As a result, they will become more sensitive and receptive to the vibrations of the higher realms.[2] By moving into higher frequencies, a physical, emotional, and spiritual transformation occurs as individuals evolve beyond what they used to be through anchoring layers of Light into the physical body. Thus raising and expanding your consciousness raises your own personal energy vibration signature.

Ascension is the name used for this expansion process whereby all humanity begins to integrate the new and higher ways of living with the new energies now available on the planet. Through the free will of the individual, the release of the accumulation of self-created negativity, and the focused effort to raise and sustain one's vibrations in a state of harmony, peace, and love, a person can achieve Ascension.[3] The goal of Ascension is to raise one's vibratory frequency to such a level of consciousness that it merges with the I AM Presence.

Ascension in the context of spiritual and planetary evolution is the natural outcome of merging our energy fields into complete and perfect alignment. The more intense and pure the alignment, the more intense and pure will be the energies that move through us while on this plane of existence.[4] According to esoteric teachings, there are seven realms (also called planes and spheres) of existence. These realms are often depicted as lying one above the other like shelves in a bookcase. However, all the realms interpenetrate.[5] These planes in order of their density are the Physical realm, the Etheric realm, the Astral realm, the Mental realm, the Buddhic realm, the Atmic realm, and the Logoic realm. In the process of ascension, we as spiritual beings will experience, purify, and master all of the realms.[6] Ascension means the elevation of consciousness and the development of a Light Body. Spiritual evolution can be challenging for many. As you move higher up the ascension ladder, you release what no longer serves you in the higher octaves. Ascension is a *process* and not an event. It is the process of raising the frequency of all the energy in the four lower bodies that include the cells of your physical body. You need a physical body that can sustain the energy to increase the vibrations of your auric bodies so you can hold the space for what is happening on the planet. This is a continual process of increasing and sustaining higher frequencies of energy. All of us have incarnated on Earth so we can be totally awakened to live from our Heart Center. In order to achieve this goal, we may need assistance to clear away any blocks to our path there. The process is different for everyone.

It would be beneficial for each of us to assess the mental prison we have constructed for our self. What are the bars holding us in our personalized prison? Are they beliefs, attitudes, and judgments? Do they really belong to us or have we absorbed them from our family and culture? Each of us has a unique style of behavior, with qualities that are both positive and negative. As we progress on our spiritual path, we eventually realize that the door to our mental prison was open all the time.

Now is the time to redesign our inner diagram. Instead of feeling helpless with the plight of being trapped in a prison of habits, it is time to focus beyond the bars and envision possibilities to escape our self-imposed bonds. Since every type of behavior and every individual is different, there is no standard timetable for change. All that is needed is a willing attitude and the desire to change. Then assume responsibility for your behavior. This includes owning your problems and taking full responsibility for your future—i.e., no longer blaming others. Once you've accepted this responsibility, you need to develop a plan of action that brings about the necessary changes, improvements, and healthy behaviors. No one else can do it for you.

Ascension Symptoms

Ascension symptoms occur because you have informed the Universe that you desire for your vibrations to be raised, and that affects the energy making up your electromagnetic fields. Becoming your True Self is your higher calling as you navigate from the third dimension of duality to the fifth dimension of Unity. Between these two dimensions is the fourth dimensional realm of the Astral Plane of emotions such as fear, anger, sadness, guilt, and anxiety. Once you become heart-centered, this Astral Plane becomes a bridge into the higher dimension of Unity Consciousness.

Your consciousness is now shifting gears from one reality to another. At the same time, you are becoming aware of the multidimensional Universe. Consequently, your human perception of time and space will be changing. The process of spiritual evolution is a personal journey and is subtle by nature as the new energies shift your four lower bodies to raise your vibratory rate. Besides the physical body, this affects the subtle bodies (etheric, emotional, and mental) that are non-physical energy bodies superimposed upon the physical body and together form the aura. These bodies are not visible to the eye, and each subtle body has its own set of chakras. Once you release all your illusions, an acceleration of vibrations occurs. This process has an upward momentum. The sooner you surrender to the symptoms of Ascension, the more quickly you will experience a rhythm and flow in your spiritual unfoldment.

Usually the Ascension symptoms challenge you in the most vulnerable areas of your life. Confronting these challenges head-on will ultimately make you stronger and more committed to the path of spiritual attunement you have chosen for this incarnation. Of prime importance, it is vital that you consult your physician to verify that there is not a medical condition associated with your physical, emotional, and mental symptoms. Many people will go to their doctor or healthcare professional, who can find nothing wrong. All the tests come back normal, and even after the second or third opinion is sought, orthodox medicine/therapies say that all is fine. Our current third-dimensional medical system is not equipped to handle these strange symptoms, and is often unable to even answer questions.[7]

There are no medical tests or conclusive measures that can let us know when our illness/ailment is a Light Body symptom. If you are experiencing unusual physical symptoms that are alarming, incapacitating, or that you feel concerned about, it is important first to consult with your medical or healthcare professional before seeking alternative holistic advice. Even if your ailment has been diagnosed as a medical condition, the effects of expanding spiritual Light will be playing a part in the manifestation of your symptoms. It is extremely important always to pay attention to your inner guidance.

The following list is an overview of the many signs and symptoms of Ascension Stress. The challenging symptoms are temporary. The key is to return to balance. Since the process of increasing the vibratory rate of each individual is different, this is not a complete list.

- Feeling stressed
- Transient body aches
- Nightly awakening between 2 and 4 AM
- Short-term memory loss
- Periods of deep sleeping
- Changes in meditation

- Inflammation, rashes, and eruptions
- Seeing or hearing things
- Relationships change
- Night sweats and hot flashes
- Intensification of your senses of sight, hearing, touch, and smell
- Unexpected flare-up of an old chronic illness
- Quicker manifestations
- Changes in energy levels
- A sense of sadness or loneliness
- Affinity for animals and nature
- Feeling joyful
- Burning sensation in the small of your back
- Increased intuitive abilities
- Feeling of pressure within the head
- Suppressed emotions emerge
- Erratic shifts in energy levels
- Attunement to the seasons, the phases of the moon, and weather patterns
- Altered states of consciousness
- Crying episodes with no apparent reason
- Heart palpitations or a dull ache between your shoulder blades
- Changes in weight and eating habits
- A sense that at some level you are different
- Increased sensitivity to environmental toxins
- Sinus and ear problems
- Feelings of being overwhelmed
- Forgotten memories resurface unexpectedly
- Feeling more supported by the Universe
- Days of extreme fatigue
- Anxiety or panic with a sense of your life being out of control

- Inner peace and a deep knowing that you are living your purpose
- Digestion disturbances
- Increased sensitivity to energies and EMFs
- Thinking you might be losing your mind
- Frequent fearfulness
- Easily overstimulated by crowds, noises, TV, and chaotic music
- Sensations of vibrations, tickling, or itchiness on top of the head
- Feeling you don't belong here and wanting to return home
- Loss of appetite
- Disorientation in time and space
- Apathy and lethargy
- Feeling angry, confused, irritable, and impatient
- Questioning life and why you are here
- Brief periods of weakness
- Erratic emotions of extreme highs and lows
- Disinterest or intolerance for lower-vibration, third-dimension situations
- Only vague remembrances of your past
- Have a higher awareness and perception of situations
- Numbness and feelings of electricity moving through your body
- Sudden disappearance of friends, activities, interests, jobs, and habits
- Difficulty doing anything that no longer matches your vibration
- Active and intense dream states
- Depression or despair
- Recalling training or initiations occurring in your dream state
- Desire to be in the presence of only like-minded people
- Suddenly develop an interest in tools of divination or healing modalities

- New food intolerances
- Occasional diarrhea for no apparent reason
- Electrical or prickly sensations in the area of the chakras
- Feeling disconnected from friends and family
- Realization of your life's purpose
- Experiencing a sense that we are all connected
- Warm palms or feet
- Higher awareness of other dimensions
- A sense of urgency to understand who you truly are
- May have conscious and spontaneous out-of-body experiences
- Strong urge to spread awareness with others to assist with their growth
- May suddenly be able to communicate with other Beings
- Dreams may be more spiritual in nature
- Intense fear of separation and loss
- Tingling in arms, hands, legs, and feet
- Back and neck spasms
- Obsessive fear of persecution and betrayal
- Emotional surges
- Respiratory discomfort, tightness in the lungs
- Dizziness, problems with coordination and balance
- Dissatisfaction with your current life
- Asthma or flu-like symptoms
- Transitory blurred vision
- Dreams or visions of past lives that can be disturbing
- Reluctance to continue in your life the same way as before
- Inflammation or aching of bones and joints
- Blood pressure instability—high or low
- Hay fever, colds, runny nose, frequent sneezing

- Life seems more effortless
- Can easily pick up the feelings, thoughts, and needs of others
- Improved understanding about how everything is connected
- Choosing to live in the moment with more ease
- No longer taking things personally
- Less desire to make things happen
- Do not care about what other people think of you
- Disinterest in mental and analytical processes
- Being more heart-centered
- An inner knowing that all needs are met and always will be

Managing Ascension Stress

The first line of defense when you are undergoing stressful situations is to focus on your physical health. Most of us know the basic strategies: make sure you acknowledge your body's sleep requirements; pay attention to nutrition choices; drink plenty of water to flush out bodily toxins; take time to experience some form of relaxation on a daily basis; and exercise daily. However, what can a person do when none of these makes a noticeable difference?

One of the keys to any type of change or healing situation is to recognize what needs to be different. Simply an acknowledgment that your present life is not working as you desire is very important. This is not an easy task for most, as it requires a deep search within the core of one's Being. Once there, you must accept that you are off track with your soul's purpose. After the awareness has been developed and accepted, it is time to form a strategy for healing and recovering. This is definitely a process. It took time to reach this state of realization, and it will take time to unwind the emotional ball of yarn that was created. Please remember that this is a journey to wholeness, and that the journey is one of the goals.

Are you aware that stress actually serves a purpose in your life? The body's reaction to a stressful condition is a physiological manifestation of the basic survival instinct. This physical process prepares you to deal with any crisis by fortifying your body with increased adrenaline. Stress can also keep your life interesting and challenging. The tricky part is to discover how to maintain equilibrium. Follow your heart and intuition and trust what resonates with you.

The whole experience for this incarnation is a lifelong process of growth and development that is ongoing until we make our final transition. We are vacillating between third-dimensional and fifth-dimensional consciousness. As such, we are slowly adapting to the elevated frequencies, so our physical body does not become overloaded. Each of you is adjusting to this transitory time at a different pace, according to your Divine Plan, for your highest and greatest good, and after many incarnations.

As the vibrations of the Earth have been increasing, so have the vibrations of the individuals on the planet since we are all interconnected. Our advancement in frequency means advancement in consciousness. Dr. David Hawkins, a well-known psychiatrist and physician, researched for twenty years and developed a method to calibrate the full spectrum of the levels of consciousness that he calls the Map of Consciousness. Dr. Hawkins discovered that consciousness vibrates at whatever frequency our thoughts and feelings vibrate. Dr. Hawkins's scale is from 0 to 1000. Zero to 20 on the scale reflects shame. Love vibrates at 500, and Enlightenment is 1000. Dr. Hawkins states that most of humanity vibrates below 200. However, he also brought forth the illuminating information that consciousness vibrating at higher frequencies has a counterbalancing effect on the lower frequencies. In addition, he discovered that it takes far fewer people vibrating in the higher frequencies to counterbalance great numbers of those who are holding a lower frequency. If you have not yet read his book *Power vs. Force: The Hidden Determinants of Human Behavior,* I strongly recommend that you do so. It will become a great addition to your reference library.[8]

The energy of the Earth and that of the people on the Earth are closely tied. Since people are not balanced in their lives, much of their release results in inappropriate behavior. A higher vibrational level means that low-frequency vibrational patterns or blockages are released at an accelerated rate. This has resulted in massive releases all over the world among people. At this point in time, soon people will have to make a choice to either move to a higher vibrational level with the Earth or to leave the Earth plane entirely.

Due to the shift into Unity Consciousness that has been flooding the Earth, all who live here are being energetically affected in some manner. The mass consciousness is vacillating on a moment-to-moment basis between embracing duality or embracing Unity Consciousness, and this instability is not easy for anyone. Be aware that the new energy pulsations are creating havoc on the Earth plane and triggering considerable anger, fear, and anxiety. If you are challenged by the symptoms of this ascension transition, try the Violet Fire techniques (Chapter 6) and the Spiritual Power Tools (Chapter 7) within this book freely and daily in your life.

A primary step in coping with the ascension process is to reframe your outlook about the ascension stress you are experiencing. Begin to view it as a blessing, since it is alerting you to a problem in your life stream. It all signifies change of some manner. Accept it as an adventure. This is one of the main reasons you chose to incarnate on this planet at this auspicious time in the history of spiritual evolution. Everyone on the planet right now is involved with ascension as each physical body adjusts to a new and higher state of existence.

Next, concentrate on the breath. This will energize you, help you focus, decrease pain perception, and assist you in relaxing more deeply. Let your awareness be completely on the breath and follow its movement. Breathe in slowly through your nose. Breathe out with lips slightly parted, tip of tongue in the groove behind your teeth at the floor of the mouth. Breathe in evenly and deeply to the count of seven. Then exhale at your own pace, tapering to a peaceful, empty pause. Feel the moment of stillness after the exhalation. Breathing this way is a gateway to peace and relaxation.

Another tool for mastering ascension stress is to make a point of doing something each day that brings you joy and leaves you energized and refreshed. One example is to take time to be with nature. The energies of nature are easily absorbed and transformed by the body. Being in nature is balancing and cleansing to your aura.[9] Awareness of the sky and seasonal changes can help open the mind for relaxation, as can the various colors in your immediate environment.

When your body's ecology is out of balance due to stressful circumstances, it is vital that you have available the types of sensory options that can help you quickly gain equilibrium. Developing a healthy relationship with your body is key. Each of us is unique, so there is no one treatment that would be universally effective for all the aforementioned ascension symptoms. The best way to navigate this time is to avoid resistance and follow the flow of energy. Trust that this process is intended to support your evolutionary growth and that the destination will be truly worth the journey. Most importantly, keep in mind there is a global spiritual awakening taking place simultaneously of unprecedented significance. The Earth itself is involved in this ascension process as it undergoes the upward spiral of its evolvement. As we move into higher states of being and into the higher realms, we are doing so through the Earth itself.

There are a number of options for you to navigate through the ascension process to restore balance and address any disharmony. Movement moves any stuck chi, so stretch, walk, jog, dance, rebound, Zumba, or do some yoga. Also, sitting and doing deep abdominal breathing for ten minutes is a form of inner movement and can reduce stress. Whenever you become fearful, angry, depressed, or shut down, just move your muscles. This will assist you in moving through the stagnation of stuck patterns instead of continually repeating them. Take the time to tune into your body and notice the emotions or feeling states that are there. Mentally ask your Body Elemental (see Chapter 12) for help to ease any aches, pains, or worry, and listen to your body to find out what it wants or needs. Perhaps it will be a warm bath, or a color, or a nap. Symptoms may ease while listening to some uplifting music or a relaxing guided meditation.

You can also quickly reverse the effects of stress by employing sensory input that brings you back into balance. By utilizing the five senses you can soothe, comfort, and energize yourself. If you react to stress by becoming shut down, depressed, or spaced out, it will be most beneficial for you to move and get active. Try going for a brisk walk, dancing to upbeat music, Qigong, doing a few yoga stretches, or some jumping jacks. Anything that will move the stagnant chi through your body and release stresses held there would be beneficial.

If you are a person who is visual, it will be best for you to surround yourself with relaxing images such as physically going to a garden, a park, or a beach. It is also effective if you just visualize the beauty of nature in your mind's eye and incorporate each of your five senses in your visualization. If you are an auditory person, it will be helpful for you to listen to uplifting music or chants as well as recordings of nature (soundtracks of the sea or forest). If you tend to become agitated under stress, try surrounding yourself with aromas that are soothing and calming. Smell flowers or utilize flower essences such as lavender and rose: spritz the essences on a light bulb, light a scented candle, or burn some incense.

For your sense of touch, you can soak in a hot tub or bath, get a relaxing massage, or snuggle with a loved one, a pet, or a favorite comforting item. By experimenting with different sensations, you can discover a variety of sensory tools that will enable you to handle any stressful situation. Chanting and singing bring joy into the body and facilitate connection to the higher realms. Listening to Gregorian chants, Tibetan singing bowls, Solfeggio Frequencies, or other ancient or sacred sounds assists in changing your frequencies. It is very helpful to develop a support system of like-minded individuals, perhaps joining a group or community to share ideas and experiences. Re-evaluate your friends and acquaintances, and surround yourself with positive and supportive people. Locate a spiritual mentor or coach to provide you with direction. To stay in your heart, pay it forward whenever possible. Lastly, pray, meditate, and ask for inner guidance about how to relieve unpleasant symptoms.

Remedies for Ascension Symptoms

There is a plethora of modalities to assist you in maintaining a level of homeostasis within your physical body during the temporary and stressful challenges of experiencing ascension. Many have been implemented by alternative health practitioners for centuries. A few are suggested below:

Whenever you become energetically stressed, drink more water and try to drink half your body weight in milliliters. Drinking revitalized and/or blessed water can nourish and nurture you. Drinking hot water with lemon upon arising can assist the body in removing toxins.

Ginger tea is useful for episodes of nausea, as is inhaling peppermint oil, which is also helpful for headaches.

Chinese Acupuncture can balance your many meridians (energy channels), calm your mind, and increase your energy in these exhausting times. It has been revered and implemented for more than seven thousand years.[10]

The Emotional Freedom Technique (EFT) is a helpful way to release negative thinking, charged emotions, and core belief patterns, all of which come up to be cleared during spiritual evolution. Instructions for this simple and effective process can easily be found online, including manuals, e-books, and YouTube videos.

Listening to a spiritual teacher or a channeled message and participating in satsangs or a guided meditation can be very comforting during a fast-moving excursion into higher consciousness. On YouTube you can find most anything.

Take frequent rest periods and short bouts of exercise, and perhaps experiment with new ways of physical activity or dance that you have never tried before.

Changes in dietary consumption can also be very effective. Juice frequently, eat foods representing all colors of the rainbow, and make alkaline food choices. An alkaline, raw, and organic diet is optimum. Avoid as much processed food as possible. Bless your food before you begin eating.

Try to avoid synthetic anything. Slowly begin to purchase and wear clothing with natural fibers like cotton, hemp, and silk.

Wear or carry crystals and gemstones that enhance your electro-magnetic field and raise your vibration. To balance the crown chakra, wear the color purple or violet and meditate with clear quartz crystal, amethyst, and lapis. Many spiritual stones are listed in Chapter 7, "Spiritual Power Tools."

Be in nature as much as possible, and plant flowers, herbs, and vegetables around your home. Place fresh flowers in your home frequently.

Be non-judgmental of others and, most of all, yourself. Remember, you are "under construction." You are no longer where you once were, but not yet where you will ultimately be.

Protect yourself from potentially harmful radiation when using cell phones, computers, and tablets. There are a number of tools available to carry or wear if you search the internet.

Cleanse and purify often. Taking a bath or shower releases stress from the body. If you are still in the workforce, it is a good idea to shower when you return home from work. As you do, visualize any negativity in your auric field swirling down the drain as the shower cascades over your body.

Drink herbal teas. University of Maryland Medical Center research shows that the menthol in peppermint tea helps relax tight muscles and improve circulation to the digestive tract. This can ease headaches and calm indigestion in as little as twenty minutes.[11]

You can reduce inflammation by eating more anti-inflammatory foods and spices such as berries, cherries, and red grapes; dark leafy greens; cruciferous vegetables such as broccoli and cabbage; black, green, and white tea; and ginger and turmeric. A more comprehensive list can be found by researching anti-inflammatory food on the internet.

According to Stanford University researchers, marjoram essential oil is a powerful anti-inflammatory that soothes sore muscles in as little as five minutes. You can make your own aromatherapy treatment by mixing 25 drops of marjoram essential oil into 8 ounces of any unscented lotion.[12]

Listen to your intuition, or dowse, as to which practitioners to choose to assist you with any mental, spiritual, or physical healings.

Avoid skin hunger by getting regular healthy touch or bodywork. If you are an energy worker, arrange frequent trades with others in your field. The constant emotional releases of the ascension process often take their toll on the physical body and even throw it off balance. That is why bodywork therapies are so vital to everyone who is spiritually progressing.

Trusting the ascension process will allow your inner knowing and physical body to better assimilate the energy shifts necessary for your transformation.

Mentally reframing the ascension process to unfold with gratitude and appreciation for the outcome will assist you in achieving a higher level of consciousness. Remember that your physical body is assisting you by holding Light as you move forward spiritually.

The fastest way to change where you are is to do something physical. Bring your dominant hand overhead and then move it vertically down the front of the body, instantly aligning the physical, etheric, emotional, and mental bodies. According to Jonathan Goldman in his book *Chakra Frequencies,* there is an astral body three to four feet from the physical body, a causal body about four to five feet from the physical body, and the spiritual body that serves as the Higher Self.[13]

Laughter is good for the soul. You may enjoy watching a comedy show to lighten your mood.

Recite certain prayers, mantras, or decrees that give you strength. Ask Source/God to align you with your soul purpose and life mission. Know and affirm that All is in Divine Order.

A particularly rewarding ritual you can employ is to bless and/or give thanks for your food before a meal. This is another method to focus your mind on gratitude. In addition, it can be very beneficial to pay attention to the present moment as you eat. By practicing mindfulness as you eat, you will slow down and focus on the smell, textures, colors, and taste of your meal. When eating slowly, you give your brain time to register that you are full, so you will likely eat less. This can allow you to have fewer digestion problems and assist in maintaining a healthy weight.

Employing essential oils is highly recommended. Use aromatherapy essential oils such as lavender, clary sage, frankincense, sandalwood, chamomile, bergamot, jasmine, and ylang ylang to relieve tension. Other essential oils can be helpful in the following specific ways:

- Muscular aches and pains: eucalyptus, rosemary, sage
- Insomnia: camphor, jasmine, marjoram
- Headaches: peppermint, lavender, cardamom, rose
- Indigestion: bergamot, fennel, lemon, peppermint

Along with relieving tension, using essential oils can enhance your immune system and remove toxins. Place a small amount of the essential oils (mixed with a carrier oil if you are sensitive) on your feet, hands, and thymus daily. During such a spiritual growth period as ascension, the body goes through a transformation process as it catches up to the shifts you've made on a soul level. It is a good time to harmonize your fears and convert them into acceptance and forgiveness. Be gentle with yourself. Take naps when you are tired, sleep late if you can, and say "no" to activities that feel restricting or drain your energy level.

Maintaining calmness in the midst of this energetic ascension chaos takes courage and commitment to shift things. You must be creative and willing to try a variety of options in order to rise above the challenges of ascension symptoms. Remember, though, they are temporary and soon you will reap the benefits.

Heart Chakra Meditation

The following is a method for allowing the body to relax and giving the mind an opportunity to gain a new perspective.

- Find a quiet, comfortable place and position.
- Take three deep breaths while closing your eyes.
- Imagine that your spine becomes longer and more elastic.
- Visualize yourself enveloped in a golden soothing circle of warmth and protection.
- Focus your awareness on your physical heart on the left side of your chest.
- Take a few deep breaths in and out in a relaxed manner.
- Breathe in as if your heart were a mouth that fills you with golden warmth and Light. Allow yourself to feel your entire body filling up with this warmth and Light.
- As you breathe in, imagine that you are inhaling all the qualities that you desire.
- Breathe in peace, tranquility, joy, love, harmony, and balance. As you exhale, release all doubts, anger, fear, sadness, worries, or concerns.
- Continue to breathe in the warmth, Light, and positive attributes and to exhale troublesome feelings, thoughts, and imbalances.
- Now ignore your thoughts and just concentrate on your breathing and the warmth and Light.
- When you are ready, slowly count from one to five and gently open your eyes.

Continued practice of this short meditation leads to cumulative benefits; however, it is best to avoid this practice when you are tired.

Chapter 3

Elimination of Barriers

Growing spiritually is no easy task and it doesn't occur overnight. Many times, our spiritual journey is filled with obstacles. These barriers can be on a physical level, psychological level, or spiritual level all thwarting out spiritual evolution. These barriers can be anything that stands in our way of reaching our goals, finding inner peace, connecting with Source, or discovering our purpose. It is important to identify what is keeping you from moving forward. Spiritual growth is a choice and cannot be achieved without going outside of your comfort zone. You have to make a conscious effort to move past your fears and doubt. The following impediments can throw us off balance and cause us to leave our spiritual practices.

Trouble Sleeping

Sleep is invaluable and provides a much-needed period of rest for the conscious mind. During sleep, the spiritual nature is allowed some freedom, much like a prisoner being released on parole. Persistent lack of sleep has a cumulative disruptive effect on your health. Sleep is essential for organ detoxification and hormone balance. How much sleep do you really need? Experts generally recommend seven to nine hours a night for healthy adults.[1]

According to well-known health advocate Dr. Joseph Mercola (see his website at www.mercola.com), there are many factors that influence the amount and/or quality of an individual's sleep. He offers thirty-three ways to optimize one's sleep experience. The following ten suggestions come from his list.

1. *The bedroom isn't dark enough.* Dr. Mercola states that the smallest amount of light can disrupt the pineal gland's production of melatonin and serotonin, which then interrupts the sleep cycle. He recommends that one close the bedroom door, use a sleep mask, and remove any nightlights. He believes that complete darkness is the best.

2. *Exercising prior to sleep.* Per Dr. Mercola, it is best to not exercise within three hours of your bedtime or it may disrupt your sleep.

3. *Consuming alcohol before bedtime.* Dr. Mercola contends that the initial drowsy effect is fleeting and the alcohol consumption can keep you from entering the deeper, restorative stages of sleep.

4. *An overly warm bedroom.* Studies show that the optimal room temperature for sleep is between 60 and 68 degrees. Since your body temperature is reduced about four hours after you are asleep, it is believed that a cooler bedroom will be more conducive to promoting sleep. You can identify the best room temperature for yourself by trial and error.

5. *Avoid caffeine late in the day.* For some, caffeine (in a beverage or medication) is not well metabolized and can hinder people from falling asleep. Avoid this substance by late afternoon.

6. *Checking the clock if you wake.* By watching the clock if you wake up in the middle of the night, you can become anxious and frustrated, which can keep you from easily resuming sleep. Dr. Mercola suggests that you move the clock to a position where it is more difficult to view.

7. *Viewing television to assist with sleep.* According to Dr. Mercola, the artificial lighting from the television (as well as computers, tablets, and readers) can disrupt melatonin

production and further delay sleep. He recommends that you avoid them at least an hour prior to sleep.

8. *Stress overload.* If worry, anxiety, and anger keep you from sleeping, you might consider keeping a journal by your bedside as a catharsis. Taking time to pray also can help keep your mind off stressors.

9. *Bedtime snacks.* It is best to avoid any food consumption three hours prior to retiring for the night. This practice will optimize blood sugar, insulin, and leptin levels and promote well-being.

10. *Having cold feet.* Scientists believe that wearing socks to bed reduces night waking, as our feet often feel cold before the rest of the body because they have the poorest circulation.

Dr. Mercola recommends moving electrical alarm clocks or other devices as far away from your bed as possible, preferably three feet away. Furthermore, he advocates that cell phones, cordless phones, and their charging stations should ideally be kept several rooms away to prevent exposure to any sleep-disrupting electromagnetic fields (EMFs). Make your bedroom an electronic free zone and ensure that all electronics in your bedroom are turned off prior to going to sleep.[2]

Other Sleep Remedies

The following environmental controls are additional strategies you might choose to implement in order to enhance your body's restoration via sleep.

Make certain you are regularly exercising. Exercising for at least thirty minutes per day, even in short bouts, can improve your sleep. However, it is not wise to exercise too close to bedtime or it may keep you awake.

Avoid food you may be sensitive to, especially sugar, grains, and pasteurized dairy. Sensitivity reactions can cause congestion, gastrointestinal upset, bloating, gas, and other problems. You may want to consider a melatonin supplement to aid sleep (it is a completely natural substance).

Listening to relaxation, guided imagery, or nature sounds such as the ocean, rain, or forest ambient noise can be soothing prior to falling asleep.

Read something spiritual or uplifting prior to bedtime to help you relax. Often journaling can be helpful if your mind won't turn off.

Go to bed as early as possible to avoid the "second wind" your body may have from recharging between 11 PM and 1 AM. Try a hot shower or bath and maybe a relaxing herbal tea thirty minutes before you go to bed.

It is best to try to wake up and go to bed at the same times each day, including weekends. This will encourage your body to get into a sleep rhythm and make it easier to fall asleep and get up in the morning.

In addition, go to bed fifteen minutes earlier each week until you can achieve seven to nine hours of sleep nightly. Avoid large meals within three hours of bedtime and mental stimulation before bed: no TV, phone calls, internet, or exercise.

Use essential oils such as lavender behind your ears to relax.

You can also employ a self-hypnosis technique by giving your subconscious mind a pre-sleep suggestion such as: *"I'm going to sleep easily and sleep deeply."*

The following technique I have had for more than thirty years, and the source is unknown.

Breathing for Sleep

- Lie flat on your back with your hands by your sides. Close your eyes.
- Slowly begin to inhale a complete breath through your nose. As you inhale, begin to raise your arms in an arc up and over your head.
- Continue to inhale very slowly for the count of ten or until your arms reach back above you and are stretched out over your head.

- Hold the breath for ten counts.
- As you exhale to a count of ten, slowly return your arms in the arc until they are resting alongside your body.
- Repeat the exercise ten times.
- Go to sleep.

With each inhalation you will begin to fall deeper and deeper into an almost dreamlike state. By lifting your arms over your head as you breathe, you give your lungs the chance to expand fully and take in a larger supply of oxygen. This increased oxygen is invaluable for quieting nerves and producing a deep and restful sleep. The "Breathing for Sleep" exercise not only can solve the difficulties of falling asleep, but it can also prepare the body for a deeper and richer sleep. If at first you cannot fulfill the count of ten, breathe in five, hold five, and release five. Gradually work your way up to a count of ten.

Dealing with Entities

Astral entities can be attracted to us via traumatic events such as catastrophic illness, loss of a spouse or child, war, psychological shock, or abuse that we may have experienced in this lifetime or others. Stressful situations such as these misalign our energy field and as a result open entry points for negative astral entities to access. They are also attracted to individuals by negative thoughts and emotions. Drug addiction and alcohol abuse are guaranteed ways to attract them.[3]

The term "entity" in this context refers to a non-physical presence that becomes an energetic parasite when it attaches to a human form. An entity is often a person who has passed on but was unable (or unready) to connect with his or her Higher Self and has remained inappropriately and unhappily with the physical plane. After the attachment to a living person occurs, the entity can create various emotional, mental, and physical problems for the host individual as well as generate voices in the head of the host.[4]

The existence of dark forces is emphasized by many world religions: Hinduism, Buddhism, Christianity, Islam, and others. Since entities have the ability to draw information from a person's memory, they can appear different in various cultural and religious contexts. Many people with an entity can at times engage in some imaginary dialog with it. However, this is more of an exchange of thoughts, as the thoughts and desires of an attached entity are experienced as the person's own thoughts and desires—for example, food cravings. An entity attachment interferes with a person's consciousness by influencing many of the person's choices and decisions. The entity becomes a mental parasite in the mind of the host and often enjoys the host's thoughts, emotions, habits, and desires, but this is quite different from hearing voices. Only a small percentage of entities manifest in the form of voices. Therefore, entity attachment must be differentiated from psychotic episodes in which individuals claim to be harassed by spirits or dark forces.[5]

There is a duality established in the Universe from the beginning. This explains the presence of the lower-density, fear-based, evil, and malevolent emotions and energies that we know on the Earth plane. Once these energies are released from their hold in the confines of the Earth, they are readily available to latch onto similar vibrations so they can feed and sustain their level of density and oppression. The healing of this beautiful planet begins with releasing entities one person at a time.

Virtually all traditional cultures considered entities real and developed methods to deal with them. Shamanic teachings, Native American traditions, Chinese Medicine, the Vedas, and the New Testament all have references to and methods of entity clearing. Since our modern Western culture disregards the existence of entities, there are very few qualified therapists trained to handle entity attachments. Generally speaking, most entities are not demonic or evil. They are an energy without an identity and thus they function as energetic parasites. Usually entities just want to survive. In most cases, entities try to conceal their presence so they can stay snug inside their host and enjoy the host's life force, emotions, and indulgences.

Occasionally mind fragments of living people can scatter due to trauma and are sometimes discovered as entities attached to another individual, carried around in a piggyback fashion.

Sometimes this situation presents itself as a subpersonality of the host.[6]

Entities often enjoy the host's desires, sensual gratification, and use of drugs and all forms of intoxication. Their influence is insidious. They send impulses such as thoughts or desires to the person's psyche that are accepted by the individual more like compulsive desires than spoken messages. So, entities do interfere with a person's consciousness by influencing their choices, decisions, and level of self-esteem. On a non-physical level, entities can be perceived as dark patches or shadows in a person's energy field. The same entity may appear differently to different people since entities exist on a level of consciousness where shapes aren't fixed.

Entities have a chameleon nature. Once you identify an entity, it will try to convince you that you can't live without it, or that it is so powerful that there is no possibility of ever getting rid of it. The reason is simple. If you release the entity, it loses its life-support system. Consequently, when someone consciously gets in touch with the entity, the entity will do everything to maintain its existence and manipulate answers to questions asked of it.

It is not advisable to perform the Entity Clearing process below for yourself unless you are familiar with working with energies from other dimensions and know how to protect yourself. If you attempt to remove spirits or entities from someone else's body or aura and do not adequately establish special protection for yourself, you could experience a psychic attack.

At this present juncture of the Earth's planned ascension, it is important to assist this energy so it can be "requalified" in the Light. This term refers to the fact that whatever a person thinks and does "qualifies" his or her energy in the sense that it imprints mental energy with either a positive or negative pattern. Energy becomes qualified or requalified spiritually due to its vibratory rate. By sending negative energy into the Light, the atoms and molecules can be charged with radiant and harmonious energies that change the rate of oscillation. If the molecular energy is not raised in this manner then it remains dense and misqualified and of a lower vibration.

The various forms of negative energy have different attributes. The higher the source of negative energy, the more "skills" the entity has developed to avoid being released.

There are dark entities that can attach to and move into physical bodies and auras, affecting what people think, speak, do, and feel. Often the human who is invaded can take on the physical attributes, illnesses, and behavior of the entity occupying or attached to them. Energy cannot die. It can only transform.

Often troubled entities (who were troubled people) stay to themselves, but they can influence and rarely even possess a person, with that person's unconscious invitation. People whose auras are open, as with alcohol, drugs, or difficult emotions, are the most frequent target for entity attachments. Someone being influenced by an entity changes noticeably, either steadily or intermittently. Sometimes there is a complete personality change as a result.

Situations that weaken our auric field and can collapse the natural human defense system include shocks and traumas, prolonged debilitating physical illness, general anesthetics, drugs, and alcohol intoxication.

Entities often need our assistance to connect with the Light and their divinity, and to move on to a happier realm. Entity healing can be a great service for your loved ones and others who have passed, for anyone being influenced, and for the Earth.[7] If you suspect that there may be a spirit attachment, you can release it with the following technique. Once again, it is not advisable to perform the following Entity Clearing process for yourself unless you are familiar with working with energies from other dimensions and know how to protect yourself. If you attempt to remove spirits or entities from someone else's body or aura and do not adequately establish special protection for yourself, you could experience a psychic attack.

This Clearing process was shared with me, decades ago, by the late Erik Berglund, who did not disclose to me its origin.

Entity Clearing

State the following *aloud*. The repetition invokes the Power of Three.

God Bless You, Energy. Thank you for all your service and the lessons you have taught. Now you are no longer needed. It is time for you to go to the place that is right for you to go at this time. I now call forth Archangel Michael and all his legions; Archangel Michael and all his legions; Archangel Michael and all his legions. At the count of three, I ask you to escort this energy to the place that is right for it to go at this time.

One...

Two...

Three....

Clap your hands and say *"BE GONE!"*

Next, visualize the entire area surrounded by Violet Fire within, around, and through wherever the entity was residing. Imagine everything filled throughout with the Violet Fire (see Chapter 6).

Ask Archangel Michael to cut away any remaining thought-forms or energy cords from the entity that was just released. Then visualize all the colors of the rainbow individually moving through the entire area and running through every object. The color order is: Red, Orange, Yellow, Green, Blue, Indigo, Violet.

According to one of my now-deceased teachers, Dr. William Baldwin, entities often described to him how they moved into an individual from behind, through the head, neck, shoulders, or back.[8] Therefore it is very important that the rainbow colors totally surround the individual.

Close with a prayer of gratitude for all the Beings who assisted you with this entity release.

Please note: You will need to repeat this process three times (speaking aloud) for each entity that is being released; or keep repeating until you, or the individual with the attachment, feels relief and/or peace.

Lack and Limitation

One important method for improving your financial abundance is to release yourself from the invisible shroud of lack and limitation. Think about lack and economic limitation as you would emotional baggage that is attached to you energetically at your physical, etheric, emotional, and mental bodies. By consciously releasing your attachment to poverty consciousness from your four lower bodies and changing the tapes you are playing endlessly in your thoughts, you can replace limitations with opportunities and abundance.

Repeat the following statement *three times* with a sincere focus and intention:

> *I release all feelings, attitudes, beliefs, and attachments of any kind to lack and limitation of abundance in my physical, emotional, mental, or etheric bodies. From this point forward, I only accept positive thoughts that lead to positive action in regard to every choice in my life. Opportunities of abundance are flowing to me from every direction in the Universe. I am open to all these opportunities. I ask Archangel Michael to sever all psychic ties to perceived limitations. So Be It.*

Now that you have decided to release lack and limitation (scarcity) as a restriction to your abundance, you will definitely need to replace the old messages of your prior belief system that have been playing over and over in your mind with new, updated, positive versions. One way to accomplish this type of reprogramming is with affirmations. An affirmation is a strong and positive declarative statement that something is already a truth. Remember that whatever you tell yourself is what you believe. Consequently, daily affirmations of abundance would be very advantageous to employ at this time.

The following list of affirmations was given to me more than twenty years ago by one of my dear spiritual teachers, Erik Berglund, who made his transition in 2013. Unfortunately, I have no idea as to the origin of these particular affirmations if they were not created by Erik himself:

Abundance Affirmations

- I have all the money I need and more.
- I deserve to make a lot of money.
- I am now achieving my financial goals.
- I always have plenty of extra cash.
- My income goes up each month.
- I believe in my unlimited prosperity.
- I choose to live an abundant life.
- I am the source of my abundance.
- I picture abundance in myself and others.
- I am increasingly magnetic to money, prosperity, and abundance.
- I trust my ever-increasing ability to create abundance.
- I accept prosperity and abundance in my life now.
- I always have more money coming in than going out.
- I draw the abundant flow of the Universe to me.
- I am abundantly provided for as I follow my path.
- I have abundance in every area of my life.
- My prosperity helps others prosper.
- I am linked with the unlimited abundance of the Universe.
- I am financially independent and free.
- Abundance is my natural state of being and I accept it now.
- I create money and abundance through, joy, aliveness, and self-love.
- I am a money magnet.
- I am financially free.
- I make more than I spend.
- I am an unlimited Being.
- I live in an abundant Universe.
- I deserve abundance.
- I am prosperous.

- I am a success.
- Money flows in my life.

With daily application and repetition of these affirmations, you can gradually program them into your subconscious mind and inculcate them into your current core beliefs. Eventually the pattern of abundance will materialize in your life.

It is important to remember that making a positive affirmation, and then allowing thoughts of doubt or disbelief to creep into your awareness, will be counterproductive and you will not achieve anything as a result.

Frequently we have the insight and intelligence to understand the entire drama we have scripted for ourselves. It is only fear that prevents us from taking action to change our script. The fears are what keep people in a state of scarcity. The fear of success is just as much a problem as the fear of failure. The fear of the unknown is just as traumatic as the choice of remaining stuck. As you change your thoughts, you change the direction of your life. It is as simple or as difficult as that. The following prayerful intention is one method to release prior core beliefs that are now deemed outmoded. Repeat it aloud, *three times,* with emphasis.

Healing Prayer to Release Limitations

I now release all separation and limitations that no longer serve my path of Light. I release all vows of poverty and limitations that I ever made in this and past incarnations. I release all imprints, self-limiting beliefs, implants, judgments, negative thought-forms, control patterns, spells and curses, negative patterns of the human ego, illness and disease patterns, and all energies that are no longer for my highest and greatest good.

Through my I AM Presence, with my full intent, I choose to release all energies of separation, limitations, and all blockages back to the Universe. I ask for these energies to be purified and requalified into the highest form of Light.

So Be It.[9]

Additionally, you can request that all negative beliefs and patterns of lack and limitation be released from your emotional body as you sleep at night. Before you drift off to sleep, surround yourself with the three concentric bubbles of protection (blue, gold, and pink). Then ask your Higher Self for this specific action to be done. You may even wish to have verification of this cellular release via your dreams.

Fear

Fear is a product of thought: of losing, of aloneness, of insecurity. Fear is the absence of love. It distracts our thinking, can make us anxious, projects us into the future, and closes the energetic life-force flow to our hearts.

Fear is an instinctive process that enables an animal to escape its enemy, but in the human it creates a negative condition. Your emotions and your habits begin to affect the entire body. You cannot set in motion negative vibrations and think they are finished. Every vibration that is set in motion tends to manifest in the physical world in some way or another. The energy created within must be released or it will create dis-ease in the physical body. If it is harmonized by our spiritual understanding that fear is a low vibration, then the effects are eliminated. By locating fear in the physical body and then flooding it with love and Light, it will be transmuted and diverted into higher channels.[10]

Fear has so many activities in the feeling world of humankind that individuals are not aware of. Many times you may have had a resistance to things that would bless you. That resistance is the fear and uncertainty that have been registered in the emotional body, by either former experiences or suggestions in the environment around you now.

The confusion humanity is experiencing mentally as well as emotionally, especially confusion in the mind, has been placed there by disturbed and discordant feelings. The suggestion of fear is everywhere in the outer world. The medical world is saturated with it; the political world is saturated with it; and the media are saturated with it. There is scarcely an activity of your daily life that isn't driving some phase of fear and doubt at your feeling world. If you accept it, fear will come into you and cause confusion and allow destructive conditions to develop.

According to the late Rev. Judith Baldwin, spiritual counselor, artist, author, and wife of William Baldwin, fear can be summarized within three main belief categories:

1. I will not get what I want.

2. I will lose what I have.

3. There is not enough to go around.

Although you may not realize it, a considerable amount of each person's energy is engaged in a kind of fear thought. Fear is the single most effective tool of the dark side, and it is immediately followed by doubt. Without your fear, the darkness would have very little influence on you. For most of us, the most salient fears concern abandonment or death. Other fears include success, rejection, change, financial problems, failure, pain, dependency, sickness, looking stupid, and loss of love.

Fear is a universal condition. It is the great obstacle to spiritual growth. As you grow older, you learn more and more fears, so by the time you reach maturity you are loaded with them. One way to understand which fear is the most disconcerting for you is to make a list of all possible fears you have. When you are finished listing them, take a moment and place a numerical value (from one to ten) next to each fear you identified in your life, with the number representing the intensity of the fear (ten being the most intense). This exercise can be quite revealing, as some fears may be disguised in dysfunctional behaviors. Unknowns create fears. When these unknowns are regularly exposed, the fears seem to diminish and disappear. To overcome fear, first face it head-on and acknowledge it openly. It will then lose its power.

Ask yourself: "Am I thinking or fearing?" Fear is not anything like love, peace, or well-being. Consequently all worry, concern, anxiety, doubt, uneasiness, revenge, guilt, blame, and resistance can be categorized as fear. With our thoughts we are either feeding fear and thereby adding to the darkness; or we are feeding peace and love and thereby contributing to the light. It is that basic and that simple. There is no middle ground of fear.[11]

Releasing Fear

Letting Go of Fear Meditation

We all experience fear. When times are changing as quickly as they are now, a basic fear for survival can surface. This exercise is based on the idea that while we are indeed undergoing stressful times, inherent within our Being is seeded an evolutionary plan that is more wonderful than our expectations. Allow yourself to feel your fear, which is the basic fear for survival. Experience the fear as it is—as energy. Let the feeling of fear pass through your body. Now concentrate on the feeling of love. Allow the feeling of love to replace the feeling of fear. Focus on your heart center and feel it expand outward into your environment. Now feel yourself being surrounded by a pink cocoon of Unconditional Love. Notice how safe and protected you feel as the fear transforms into love.[12]

Next, declare and acknowledge to your conscious and subconscious mind that you have now developed Mastery over (name a fear). Then release it into the Universe in a hot-air balloon. Your subconscious will move on to the next experience, as it believes the former experience is now complete.

Another very effective technique to release fear is to write a letter either to your fear(s) or to the particular organ or body part that houses it. The easiest way to begin the letter is to start writing without thinking and without an agenda. Do not lift your pen from the paper. Just journal everything and anything you are currently experiencing. Then dialogue with the fear and thank it for providing protection, of sorts, to you. If you are ready, invite it to leave.

You may feel more comfortable drawing a picture of your fear or the place where you feel it lodged in your body. Draw it in vivid colors and shapes. You can also use visualization to remove the fear once you have decided it no longer serves you. Just use your imagination to give it a color, a shape, and a texture. Notice where it is stored in your body. Then with focus and intention, mentally shrink it down in size until it completely disappears.

Begin to pay attention to your dreams. Keep a dream journal and try to get in touch with your fears as they are revealed in your subconscious mind through your dream state. Eventually you will reach a point where situations no longer elicit fear. The process will be like a metamorphosis rather than a sudden about-face.

Still another method for releasing emotional blockages caused by fear is to change the program in your mind through the repetition of affirmations. Take a moment to think about yourself without your fear. Create a positive statement for each attribute you wish to develop. Then write each attribute twenty times every day. Writing these just before you go to sleep is an excellent idea. This exercise will assist you in reprogramming the computer of your mind and changing your self-concept. Lastly, you may wish to contact a therapist who specializes in hypnosis, rapid eye desensitization, or neuromuscular release to eliminate the root cause.

Your protective aura can become damaged from within by rational, habitual, or sudden fear. Rational fear is based on a real and dangerous situation. Habitual fear occurs when the fear is out of proportion to the real facts of a situation. Sudden fear is irrational and caused by subliminal influences. An example of the latter is the continual media showing of the events of a tragedy. All three of these fears can create openings in your auric field that will eventually magnetize more fear to you.

There are many techniques to strengthen your auric field against generalized negativity and psychic attacks throughout this book and especially in Chapter 5, "Spiritual Protection." Most use a visualization technique and all require a strong focus and intention to be protected from outside interferences and negativity. Experiment with these techniques until you find one or two that allow you to be buffered and protected from discord.

Lack of Self-Love

It is vital that you develop a healthy self-concept in order to progress spiritually. The ability to love begins with the ability to love yourself, right where you are now, warts and all, failures and fears. Love is your birthright. It is who and what you essentially are at the core of your Being.[13]

Before you can truly love someone, you must learn to love yourself. In fact, it's easy to see how far you have progressed along the continuum of loving yourself by reviewing the thoughts you have of others. Since other people act as mirrors for us, when we look into the eyes of another and see a loving person, we know that it is our own love that is being reflected back to us. Conversely, when we see fear, anger, or some other discordant emotion we will know that those are the issues within us yet to clear. Judgment may creep into your thoughts about another person. As you judge others, you have judged yourself, because we are all connected. It is through the Universal Mind and holographic nature of being One with All There Is that we see, sense, or feel that all that is within us is reflected back to us.

So what exactly is self-love? It is developing your creative drives; surrounding yourself with people who nourish you; having confidence in your abilities; acknowledging and praising yourself verbally to yourself; letting others in instead of submitting to loneliness; trusting yourself; forgiving yourself; creating an abundance of friends; following your intuition; seeing yourself as equal to others; giving yourself pleasure without guilt; taking credit for what you did; loving your body and seeing only its good qualities; giving yourself what you want and feeling you deserve it; becoming your own approving parent; getting a massage frequently; and turning all your negative thoughts into positive affirmations. At the end of your day, reflect on what you have accomplished and who you have touched that day, rather than focusing on what went wrong and what you didn't accomplish. It is often just a matter of programming your internal computer differently from the way that your parents or society programmed you.

Chronic Reversed Polarity

According to Master Herbalist Keith Smith, Chronic Reversed Polarity is a disease of the physical electrical system that negatively alters the body's immunity, mental health, and overall well-being. He believes that this condition is the root cause of Chronic Fatigue Syndrome and many other diseases. The body is an electrical system, and electricity flows around the body, creating an electromagnetic field. This electromagnetic field, like that of the Earth, has a north and a south pole. When something causes a shift in your system, your axis can also change. Then your poles become reversed and your body can no longer operate in an optimal manner. Stress causes your polarity to become reversed. This can be physical, mental, or emotional in nature. Car accidents, divorces, deaths, bad relationships, stressful jobs, financial issues, and other traumatic experiences are powerful enough to reverse a person's polarity and change the direction that the root chakra normally spins.[14]

Since your body is not functioning normally, it is not able to hold any healing modalities such as chiropractic adjustments, homeopathy, acupuncture, or even conventional medical treatments. In this reversed state, there is a constant pull to maintain the reversal, causing a person to relapse over and over again, no matter what treatment is implemented.

The most common symptoms are fatigue (even after a good night's sleep), difficulty sleeping, inability to focus, short-term memory loss, depression, anxiety, foggy brain, numbness and pain in the extremities, frequent illness, allergies, adrenal fatigue, weight gain, and a general feeling of debilitation. However, not all these symptoms need to be present to have Chronic Reversed Polarity. A person may have only one of these symptoms and be in Chronic Reversed Polarity.

Some of us are born into this condition. We acquire it from our parents. Some of us acquire it from our job, our lifestyle, our passions, or just plain living in today's world. Fortunately, this condition can be permanently shifted back to normal and balanced via Keith Smith's herbal program over four to six months.[15]

Unhappiness

When people experience repeated negative situations, it is easy to become bitter, cynical, and ungrateful. Since each person lives within the energy they emit into their aura, the more discordant feelings they generate, the unhappier they become. Therefore, it is best to learn to generate an aura of a happy nature, for that is the resonance in which the soul must dwell. One way to generate a state of happiness and well-being is to focus continually on your gratitude. Gratitude is the activity of loving life free from distress.[16]

Negative energy can only be dissolved or transmuted by positive energy. As soon as you hear yourself saying a negative, inappropriate, or judgmental statement, stop immediately and state *aloud: "Cancel Clear!"* This will cancel out the erroneous statement you just voiced before it can be imprinted in your subconscious mind. Then immediately replace the negative thought by saying aloud a positive statement.

Chapter 4

Clearing Your Living Space

For more than twenty-five years, I have been performing remote Spiritual Clearings for people, animals, and places. Since the procedure can be done long-distance, I don't have to physically be present during the Spiritual Clearing process. When working to change the vibrational level in a physical space, I also determine if there are physical changes that can be made to improve the basic flow of positive energy. Currently there is a plethora of books available containing proven methods for Space Clearing and Feng Shui; these provide simple "cures" that often make an immediate contribution to improving the movement of energy (chi) in a physical space.

Improvements may involve clearing away clutter, rearranging furniture, using colors and the five elements (Wood, Fire, Earth, Metal, and Water) properly in the space, or following the Bagua map. Other options would be adding color accents, plants or fresh flowers, and mirrors; burning sage or copal resin; and airing the rooms frequently. Naturally, you can always enhance positive energy with additional lighting in an area. Energies can be transformed on both a physical and energetic level.

Many people concentrate on the physical and overlook unseen or etheric energy areas. Once the physical changes have been made, etheric energy considerations must be addressed to bring all the vibrations to the appropriate level. These are not equally weighted in importance. While the physical changes are important, the energetic changes are essential.

There are many ways to change the etheric energy, and I offer several suggestions here; however, it would be impossible to address every situation without specific details. Prayer is a universal example of an ancient method to elevate the energy signature of a location. Praying in any space always increases the vibrations, and the cumulative effect of prayers in a space will inevitably create a powerful vortex. On the contrary, wherever intensely negative energies have been displayed in a space, a negative etheric vortex is created that must be dismantled before significant positive progress can be sustained.

Such a compilation of negative energies may be due to a number of factors that include (but are not limited to):

- Emotional residue from previous occupants
- Discarnate souls (discussed in Chapter 3, the section entitled "Dealing with Entities") existing in the space or attached to objects or memories
- Presence of various negative thought-forms or energies
- Geopathic stress on the property; this comes from toxic streams of energy below the ground's surface
- Electromagnetic interferences such as cell phone towers and "Smart Meters"

The Home Clearing Process in this chapter is particularly effective in removing these discordant energies, and the Violet Flame discussed in Chapter 6 is always available and helpful.

Keeping your vibrations and the vibrations of your living space elevated helps to lift the density of the immediate atmosphere. This is accomplished through intention and a daily practice of gratitude for the maximum effect. Implementing a "Blessing" for your home and property on a regular basis can shift any lower-vibrational energy that may be present. The following blessing can be simply spoken aloud or incorporated in a ceremony with candles and incense. Whichever way is chosen, it must be done with intention and gratitude. The main focus is to evoke blessings, protection, and peace for the site and all who dwell there.

These blessings can be extended to the garden, patio, or porch. Each represents a place of rest and relaxation that can lift your mind and heart to the marvels of nature. The following is an example of a simple yet powerful house blessing. The power comes through your sincerity of intention and connection with Divine will.

Dear Source of All That Is,

Please bless this home and fill it with the presence of Life, Light, Truth, Health, Purity, Prosperity, Peace, and Harmony. I ask for this home to be filled with Joy. I am surrounded by Joy. I am filled with Joy and Happiness. Whoever enters here will be conscious of the presence of Joy. Only Love dwells within this home. This home radiates Love to all who enter. All discordant energy is now cast out. Love fills these walls. Whoever enters here will be conscious of the pure, holy presence of Love.

I ask Source to bless this dwelling and fill it with your Presence. I am thankful that all who enter here will be conscious of the Presence of Source.

Amen

The turbulence of the Earth changes at the end of the last century allowed many types of accumulated and trapped negative energies to be freed from the Earth. The main purpose of these upheavals was to assist Mother Earth with the cleansing of a multitude of humanity's negative and destructive thought-forms and energies that were anchored on and within the Earth for centuries. Everything is changing, as we are all moving together into a new state of being and letting go of third-dimensional concepts. We will be unable to take these old values and ways of existing into the infrastructure of the New Earth and Unity Consciousness. This natural purging, predicted by many ancient cultures, will allow the Earth to be purified from the dense energy forms attached to Her from the beginning of time, so the Earth can ascend to the fifth dimension.

In the current world situation, it is obvious that many people are giving energy to war, oppression, disaster, control, hunger, and limiting religious beliefs. These are the same types of energies that have been stuck for the last thousand years or more and must now be released. Unfortunately, fear feeds this same kind of energy. As long as anyone remains in the same low-vibrational energy that they fear, they will remain trapped within that density.

However, once these energies are released from the confines of the Earth, they will be free to latch onto similar dense vibrations of others, much like the roaming of free radicals within our human bodies. The negative energies through their attachment to individuals, places, and things will continue to create density and oppression. We, as individual Emissaries of Light, have a responsibility to assist the Earth with this purging of negativity. The healing of this beautiful planet begins one person at a time. One good place to begin is by clearing away negative and stagnant energies within your own immediate environment. If you are interested in more specific techniques for performing a Self-Clearing, please read my book *Spiritual Clearings.*

What Is a Spiritual Clearing?

Just like bacteria, which can be discerned physically without technology, the world of energy exists as well. The Archangels and Nature Spirits (Elementals) have long volunteered to help humanity lift away the layers of unseen negativity that have accumulated on the Earth plane from wars and cataclysms. The Spiritual Clearing process I am about to share is a specific procedure for removing negativity by utilizing the assistance of the highly evolved spiritual Beings from higher realms of existence. With this Divine assistance, a strong vortex of energy is created through prayers, mantras, and affirmations. The following information about how to work in concert with these Beings of Light was provided to me decades ago during several meditations. Through the years I have found that there are many levels of negative energy in the astral plane. Each of these categories of energy must be removed separately using a unique method and spiritual assistance for that particular level. The actual release of all levels of negative energies is accomplished by the Angelic and Nature Kingdoms that are summoned to help.

Typically there is a remarkably positive change in people and animals within approximately seventy-two hours after a Home and Property

Clearing takes place. Generally the household seems less tense and stressful, children are less fearful, and people sleep better. Often people state that the property is more vibrant and the space feels more open.

Frequently, dwellings that have had a series of renters or have been on the market for a considerable amount of time are filled with stagnant and disharmonious energies and thought-forms. This is especially true of the discordant energies found in homes that are sold due to divorce. Negative energy can be left by former tenants or it can be transported to a place by workmen or visitors. After purchasing a new home and before you move in is the best time to do a Spiritual Clearing.

Other situations that would benefit from a Home and Property Clearing include:

- Real estate listings that are not moving
- Rental properties
- Dwelling was vacant for a long period
- Sites where death or abuse occurred
- Properties related to divorce or disputes
- Furnished with used furniture
- Many artifacts from foreign countries
- Decorated with antiques or heirlooms
- Rooms or areas feel creepy and are avoided
- Presence of rented convalescent equipment
- Previous occupants had a lingering illness or died in the home
- Former occupants were addicted to alcohol or drugs
- Site of frequent parties or large gatherings
- Close proximity to a cemetery, hospital, or funeral home
- Historical home or located in a historical district
- Feeling exhausted or depressed when at home, but nowhere else
- Experiencing waves of fear when home alone
- Difficulty sleeping or nightmares since moving in
- Dwelling feels haunted

- Death or illness of a pet shortly after moving in
- Behavior changes in pets since moving
- Objects frequently disappear and then reappear
- Actual sightings of an apparition
- Unusual anger or irritability since moving in
- Disputes with neighbors since moving in
- Poor concentration only when at home
- Feeling as though you were being observed
- Children are afraid to go upstairs to their bedrooms

Changing the Vibrations in a Location

The process that I require to carry out a Spiritual Clearing for a home or property may be quite different than what you expect; however, it is a far more powerful process than simply smudging an area with sage. As you will notice, the "Spiritual Clearing Team" that is summoned is composed of representatives of the Angelic and Nature Kingdoms that have volunteered to help us humans keep our environments cleared. You will also be introduced to the concept of working with the Devas, who are Nature Beings of the property and are similar to the Guardian Angels of humankind.[1]

Members of the Spiritual Clearing Team

Since many of you may be unfamiliar with the specific Beings that compose the Spiritual Clearing Team, I offer a very brief overview of the Dimensional Beings (who they are and how they are assisting humanity) who are called forth to perform the Spiritual Clearings for a home or business.

- **Master St. Germain**
  He is the Lord of the Seventh Ray of Transmutation. The nature of the Seventh Ray is to purify the energy and substance of life. His gift to humanity is the Violet Transmuting Flame that can

be invoked through the power of visualization, contemplation, intention, or by decree. It can be used to consume mistakes, remove negativity from self or environment, cleanse and purify your mind, and raise your vibrations. Chapter 6 is devoted to the topic of the Violet Transmuting Flame, also known as the Violet Fire.

- **Angels of the Violet Flame**
These are the Angels of the Seventh Ray who purify everything whenever they pass through. There are Legions of these Violet Fire Angels. When summoned, they gather around you. With palms outstretched, they direct across your four lower bodies and your aura an arc of the Violet Ray. As that arc flashes across your Being, it vaporizes the negative conditions from your heart and mind.

- **Archangel Michael**
He is known as the Archangel that battles evil and cleanses people and places of discord and negativity. His color is blue and he is the Angel of Protection. He challenges humans who hold evil or negative intentions to transmute them into positive and higher Divine energies. His Flaming Blue Sword can be called upon to sever your self-imposed psychic ties to perceived limitations and attachments.

- **Archangel Raphael**
He is known as the Archangel of Healing and the guardian of creative talents who brings happiness and joy. His color is green. He is charged with the sacred duty to heal the Earth and to heal humanity of its maladies. The staff Raphael carries (resembling a shepherd's staff) symbolizes this.

- **Archangel Uriel**
Known as the Archangel of Truth, he helps us with intellectual information, practical solutions, and creative insight. He transmutes all distortions connected with truth including lies, misuse of power, and energies related to various forms of self-deception. His colors are ruby and gold.

- **Archangel Gabriel**
  Gabriel is known as the Archangel of Mercy. He is the bringer of good news and a catalyst for change who assists people with their spiritual purpose. His color is white and his symbol is the lily.

- **Mother Earth** (also known as Gaia)
  The Earth is a Living Being whose body has many parallels to our own. It is also an electromagnetic organism that runs on energy.

- **Devas**
  These are Nature Beings, similar to the Guardian Angels of humankind, that exist in a parallel kingdom to humanity. Each deva has its specific area of responsibility to oversee.

  - **Deva of the Earth Kingdom**
  - **Deva of Dwelling** (state address or geographical location)
  - **Deva of** (the name of this city)
  - **Deva of** (the name of this state)

- **Pan and the Nature Spirits**
  Pan is the heart energy that fine-tunes the frequencies among the Elementals and Mother Earth and our personal vibrations by working with the frequencies of Love and Light. Pan exists on a universal and multidimensional level.

- **Elemental Kingdom** (Fire, Air, Water, and Earth)
  The Elementals are the nature spirits of fire, air, water, and earth who are responsible for taking care of our planet.

- **Ancestors and Guardians of** (state area or property)
  Often, the land receiving a Spiritual Clearing might still be inhabited by ancestor spirits of the original landowner or occupants. In many situations the Native American or indigenous people living in an area were removed forcibly and/or violently. By requesting the assistance of these Beings, the imprinted negative energies of these past actions can be released from the confines of the Earth.

Home and Property Clearing Process

To implement this Spiritual Clearing process, you will need a white candle (a small votive will do) and a lighter of some type. You can use a battery-operated candle if you prefer. You might also wish to have a pen and paper available in case you want to jot down some notes or experiences. Lastly, you will need to have this book or a copy of the procedure to follow. If you are skilled in any type of dowsing or muscle-testing technique, you can obtain a more specific listing of the negative influences that are present. Otherwise you can simply read each category aloud individually. This Home and Property Clearing process is designed to be read *aloud* as a script. For the most success, it is important to follow the flow as it is given here, as this process has been tested in hundreds of thousands of Spiritual Clearings. To be the most effective, do not omit any of the steps listed. Allow about forty-five minutes to an hour where you won't be disturbed to complete this Spiritual Clearing process. Remember to follow the script as it is written and read out loud everything that is printed in *bold*.

Find a place where you will be comfortable and won't be disturbed for about an hour. You may play some soft music if you wish, but please turn off your cell phone out of respect to the Beings that are assisting you with clearing your home and property. When you have everything that you might need, including a beverage, then light the candle to begin the process.

Information about the following prayer can be found in Chapter 7, in the section entitled "Favorite Prayers."

The Great Invocation

From the point of Light within the Mind of God
Let light stream forth into human minds.
Let Light descend on Earth.

From the point of Love within the Heart of God
Let love stream forth into human hearts.
May the Coming One return to Earth.

From the center where the Will of God is known
Let purpose guide all little human wills—
The purpose which the Masters know and serve.

From the center which we call the human race
Let the Plan of Love and Light work out
And may it seal the door where evil dwells.

Let Light and Love and Power
restore the Plan on Earth.

Preparation Prayer

I come in Love and Light and ask my Higher Self and Guardian Angel for guidance during this Spiritual Clearing process. I ask that only the Truth shall come through.

Protection Force Field

Dear Source,
Please surround me (and my home) in the blue bubble of Divine power,
In the gold bubble of Divine wisdom, and the pink bubble of Divine love.

Raising Vibrations

Lord's Prayer

(Repeat three times)

Our Father, Who art in heaven, Hallowed be thy name.
Thy Kingdom Come, Thy Will be done on Earth as it is in Heaven.
Give us this day our daily bread,
And forgive us our debts as we forgive our debtors.
And lead us not into temptation, but deliver us from evil.
For Thine is the Kingdom and the Power and the Glory, forever.
Amen

1. **Light Decree**

(Repeat the series three times)

Light! Light! Light!

2. **I AM Decree**

(Repeat the series three times)

I AM That I AM
I AM That I AM
I AM That I AM

3. **Soul Mantram**

I AM the Soul,
I AM the Light Divine,
I AM Love,
I AM Will,
I AM Fixed Design.

4. **Violet Fire Decree**

(Repeat three times)

I AM a Being of Violet Fire!
I AM the purity Source desires!

5. **OM**

(Repeat this mantra three times)

Invoking the Spiritual Clearing Team

I align with my Higher Self and my I AM Presence as I call forth:

- *My guides and teachers of 100% pure Light*
- *Master St. Germain*
- *Angels of the Violet Flame*
- *Archangel Michael*
- *Archangel Raphael*

- *Archangel Uriel*
- *Archangel Gabriel*
- *Mother Earth*
- *Deva of the Earth Kingdom*
- *Deva of (the name of the city)*
- *Deva of (the name of the state)*
- *Pan and the Nature Spirits*
- *Elemental Kingdom (Fire, Air, Water, and Earth)*
- *Ancestors and Guardians of (state area or property)*
- *Deva of Dwelling (state address or geographical location)*

Setting Intentions

> *I set my intention to work in harmony with the Beings of Light, Archangels, Devic Kingdom, Nature Spirits, Mother Earth, and the other energies assisting me today for the highest good of all. My intention is to bring balance, peace, and harmony to* (state exact address or geographical location).

Asking for Permission

Mentally focus or "tune in" to your heart center. Ask for permission to do a Spiritual Clearing at the specific site or area. You can ask telepathically or by dowsing with rods or a pendulum, muscle testing, or listening quietly for an inner voice. Stay neutral to the answer and remove your personal will from the situation. If the answer you intuit is a "yes," you may proceed with the Spiritual Clearing. If the answer is a "no," you will be unable to perform the Spiritual Clearing at this time. Please thank all those you have summoned for the Spiritual Clearing and release them with gratitude and love.

Encircling the Spiritual Clearing Area

> *Please encircle* (state address or area) *with White Light and permeate this circle and everything in it with unconditional love and the highest*

level of cleansing energy and increase it as needed throughout this Spiritual Clearing process. Please make this circle bigger than the area involved.

Requesting Protection

I ask the Universe to place me in the Protective Pillar of Light and to send back, on all levels and dimensions, anything and everything that is interfering with my Free Will.

Releasing Negative Energies

Read each category aloud and request that it be removed.

I request removal of all:

- *Discarnate beings*
- *Energetic residents*
- *Negative thought-forms*
- *Negative essences*
- *False beliefs*
- *Energy cords*
- *Prejudices*
- *Accumulated negative energies*
- *Astral entities*
- *Disharmony*
- *Negative elementals*
- *Vibrational influences*
- *Stagnant energy*
- *Fragmented souls*
- *Dark angels*
- *Negative emotions*
- *Energy interferences*
- *Negative frequencies*

- *Unknown dark forces*
- *All other negative influences of any type*

I ask the Universe to dissipate, dissolve, and return them all back to their source on all levels and dimensions.

Blessing the Dwelling or Property

I ask the Archangels to radiate Love into my home, the contents, and property.

You can assist by imagining every room filling with a glorious pink mist, which represents Unconditional Love.

Positioning the Deva

I ask that the Deva be placed over my home and property so it may stream Love down to envelop the entire area. I ask that my home and property now be encircled with the blue and gold and pink bubbles of protection.

Closing the Spiritual Clearing

In the name of Light, I give thanks to all the Beings who assisted me with this Spiritual Clearing today. I say thank you and Amen to:

- *My guides and teachers of 100% pure Light*
- *Master St. Germain*
- *Angels of the Violet Fire*
- *Archangel Michael*
- *Archangel Raphael*
- *Archangel Uriel*
- *Archangel Gabriel*
- *Mother Earth*
- *Deva of the Earth Kingdom*

- *Deva of* (the name of the city)
- *Deva of* (the name of the state)
- *Pan and the Nature Spirits*
- *Elemental Kingdom* (Fire, Air, Water, and Earth)
- *Ancestors and Guardians of* (state area or property)
- *Deva of Dwelling* (state address or geographical location)

Blow out the candle. Then center and ground yourself by walking outside in nature, holding some grounding stones, or visualizing a connection with the Earth.

This Spiritual Clearing is more versatile than it appears. It can be utilized to release negativity from animals, cars, books, crystals, computers, antiques, used clothing and furniture, jewelry, and foreign artifacts, to name a few. On the other hand, this process *cannot* be used for a Spiritual Clearing of a person, as that is far more complicated and takes advanced training in order to avoid absorbing another person's karma.

Chapter 5

Spiritual Protection

You would not be reading this book unless you have embraced your spiritual side and wish to develop it more fully. As you advance on your spiritual journey, it is vital that you pray and ask for protection every day, as well as create it for yourself. The protection you ask for is from all forms of negativity. There is a lot of negativity in the world at this time. As you bring forth more Light, darkness is drawn to it as if by a magnet. Make it a habit to place protection around yourself and your loved ones twice a day. It would be ideal to request spiritual protection every morning upon arising, every afternoon, and before going to bed at night. If you do this consistently, the negative invasion can be avoided considerably.[1] I also recommend that you consider performing a weekly Spiritual Clearing for yourself, as instructed in my first book, *Spiritual Clearings*.[2]

I suggest that you call upon Archangel Michael every day to place a golden dome of protection around you, especially upon awakening and, more importantly, before going to sleep. You can intercept many, many problems in your life by taking the time to do these simple spiritual exercises. It is when you get lazy and don't do them that you become vulnerable. If you own your power and create your protection, then in truth you have nothing to be concerned about.[3]

Tri-Colored Force Field Daily Protection

As part of a daily spiritual practice, visualize or imagine three protective, concentric circles around you to maximize your spiritual protection. These bubbles, also called the Bubbles of Protection, are blue (Divine power), gold (Divine wisdom), and pink (Divine love). Visualize or imagine that you are totally surrounded by a blue bubble. Around the blue bubble is the gold bubble that is surrounded by the pink bubble. In this manner, the bubble of power is closest to your body and the outer bubble is the vibration of love. This visualization takes only a few moments to do and yet it is very powerful if done on a *daily* basis, especially before sleeping and before starting the day.

Use the following prayer/intention in whatever variation is comfortable for you to say or visualize:

Dear Mother/Father God or Source,

Please surround me (and/or my home) in the blue bubble of Divine power, the gold bubble of Divine wisdom, and the pink bubble of Divine love.

Thank you.

Pillar of Light

Since we live now in the psychic realm, there are living, pulsating, negative vibrations around us. These are great clouds of emotional and mental thought-forms that move like a whirlpool of energy emanating negativity and influencing all of us. They are the causes and cores of centuries of discordant energy created by humanity and its wars, and by cataclysms and other chaotic events, and it is important that you start your day with protection from them, like the Pillar of Light.[4]

This protective pillar is a tube of pure Light substance, invisible to ordinary sight, but it can be seen with inner vision. However, it is not hollow like a tube. Rather, it has light all the way through it like a pillar in, through, and around your body, for a radius of about three (or up to nine) feet. It is like a tube composed of fiery, opaque, white spiritual fire, condensed at the outer edge, like a border, to make it impenetrable to anything not of the Light. It is charged in, through, and around the physical body. It extends from above the head to below the feet, giving protection to the inner bodies as well as the physical. See or imagine it descending from your I AM Presence and extending nine feet in diameter, all around you and beneath your feet. Imagine it blocking all negative energy directed at you. Then see the tube filled with Violet Fire, its spiritual energy freeing you from your worries and concerns.[5]

To invoke this Pillar of Light, state the following:

I call upon my I AM Presence to project, establish, and intensify your protective pillar of pure Light in, through, and around me—charged with your invincible protection, all-powerful and impenetrable, which keeps me absolutely insulated to everything not of the Light, and keep it sustained. Thank you.

No matter what responsibilities you have, throughout the day you may be bombarded with other people's fears, negative thought-forms, and excessive demands. How can you manage to stay centered and at peace in the midst of all that? Call forth the Pillar of Light to build a powerful energy of protection around you. It can insulate you from negative forces emanating from a person sitting next to you or even touching your physical body. Additionally, this technique can allow you to be disconnected from the mass-consciousness thought-forms in the atmosphere.

These thought-forms are a collection of thoughts that have been released by humanity (the collective) over the years that attract additional thoughts of the same kind. As an example, when a cataclysm occurs, there may be thought-forms of fear released by thousands of people that are real energies. These energies remain in the atmosphere and become like a huge cloud of fear for people to experience until it is released. Certain places on the Earth have denser concentrations of these thought-forms than others. Consider the Middle East and all that has historically transpired in that region. The lingering thought-forms from those past situations can still affect people today who are physically in or pass through that area.

This Pillar of Light must be created each day before starting your routine anew. It is an extension of your I AM Presence that descends in answer to your call. This cylinder of shimmering White Light keeps out negative energy and seals in the Violet Flame, thus helping you maintain your connection to your I AM Presence. It protects you from the energies of hatred, jealousy, anger, and manipulation by others about the way you should be, think, or act. It will protect you from any imperfect thought-forms that are floating in the atmosphere. If you start your day with this Pillar of Light, you can have that protection before any negativity comes your way.[6]

Though external negative energy cannot break it, the Pillar of Light can dissipate if you withdraw your attention from your I AM Presence. It can also be temporarily torn if you allow yourself to become upset. Since the stressors of your day can distract you from maintaining a constant connection to your I AM Presence, it is best to give this decree at the start of each day to re-establish this protective force field around you. Then you can reinforce it by saying the decree at various intervals throughout your day such as when driving or riding public transportation, or while doing daily chores, and focus on the image of the pillar in your mind's eye.[7]

Visualize the Pillar of Light around you. When saying the following mantra, repeat it aloud three times for the most effect.

Pillar of Light Mantra

Beloved I AM Presence bright,
Round me seal your Pillar of Light
Let it keep my Being free
From all discord sent to me.[8]

Circle of Blue Flame

If added protection is needed, invoke the following:

I ask my I AM Presence to surround my Protective Pillar of Light with your Circle of Blue Flame and provide whatever added protection is required. I thank you.

Then picture or sense this Circle of Blue Flame (about four inches thick) completely surrounding your Pillar of Light. This must also be established on a daily basis.[9]

The following two meditations for spiritual protection were created by one of my spiritual teachers, the late William Baldwin, PhD, who was a pioneer in the area of Spirit Releasement.

Inner Shrine Meditation

Sit in a chair with feet flat on the floor, your back straight, hands held out about twelve inches away, palms facing your Heart Center so energy will go toward the self.

Then visualize a Violet Flame sweeping up through your feet, swirling through the lower bodies and bathing every cell with its cleansing, transmuting power. This is a cleansing process to remove cloudiness or darkness and build the Inner Shrine.

It needs to be created every day in order to become a pure channel for Source.

- Now think of your Higher Self as a sun and visualize a Golden Light coming from this sun—like a star or flame over your head—entering through the top of your head.

- When the Light is steady and is seen (or felt) with the "inner eye," focus on the Heart Center and visualize the sparkling star as before. Now extend the Light, by thought, until you feel the energy flow slowly through your body down to the feet. You may feel a tingle or warmth.

- Next, through your intention, bring the Light back up to the heart and expand it out to the etheric body, then the emotional body, and then to the mental body—illuminating every atom.

- After cleansing and balancing the above bodies by use of the Christ Energy that flows into your crown and through your hands, fill your entire Being with sparkling Blue-White Light.

This same Light will also be used to encircle your magnetic field (which is egg-shaped). This will protect you from mass consciousness and evil thoughts directed toward you. An opening at the top will direct the Christ Light to you and protect you from all darkness.[10]

Sealing Light Meditation

According to the late Dr. Baldwin, this meditation is the first step in self-protection. It is to be visualized first thing in the morning upon awakening, several times a day, and at bedtime. After some practice, the visualized Sealing Light Meditation becomes automatic. It is like a light that is always on.

- Visualize or imagine a brilliant point of Light that is deep within your chest area. This spark of Light is your connection with Source and is always there.

- See this Light expand into your whole body. Feel the Light energy flowing through your arms and out your hands, moving down your legs and out your feet, and then filling your head.

- Now imagine that the Light is expanding out past the boundaries of your body, outside your physical form.

- Notice it expanding out to an arm's length in front of you, an arm's length behind you, and an arm's length on either side of you, as high as you can reach above your head, and down beneath your feet.

- See and feel this Light now, lovingly surrounding you like a large egg-shaped cocoon or bubble of Light.

- Sparkling through this cocoon of Light now, begin to imagine iridescent pieces of emerald green for healing and iridescent pieces of rose pink for love.

- This cocoon of Light does not interfere with any outward expression or incoming experience of love.

- Repeat this meditation of Light when you awaken and before you got to sleep.

- Also repeat this meditation whenever you feel tired or unhappy.

- See and feel this shimmering bubble of Light every time you breathe. Soon it will be with you permanently.[11]

Armor of Light

An individual can also summon an Armor of Light for protection. With your intention, imagine a golden light substance fitting closely around your body. It is similar to the ones worn by crusaders and warriors with helmets and full body coverage. Then surround it with the Circle of Blue Flame for added protection, like you can do with the Pillar of Light.[12]

Light Worker's Shield

The following is adapted from one of my spiritual teachers, the late Erik Berglund.

I ask that a Light Worker's Shield be put in place around me now.

I ask that blue *light stream within, around, and through my entire Being.*

I ask that gold *light stream within, around, and through my entire Being.*

I ask that pink *light stream within, around, and through my entire Being.*

I ask that a rainbow of colors (red, orange, yellow, green, blue, indigo, and violet) swirl within, around, and through my entire Being.

I ask that white *light stream within, around, and through my entire Being.*

I ask that blue *light form an exterior grid on the outside of this Shield.*

I ask that gold *light layer over the blue grid on the outside of this Shield.*

I ask that pink *light finalize and surround the entire outside of this Shield.*

I now ask my Higher Self to weave an Infinity Symbol of shimmering White Light around everything, and for the Universe to maximize this protection that has been created.

Chapter 6

Violet Fire

Violet Fire is a Divine energy that raises the vibration of all its contacts with a spiritually harmonizing effect. Violet Fire vibrates at the highest ultraviolet spectrum of the color frequencies and can be evoked through visualization and the spoken word. It is also referred to as the Violet Transmuting Flame. It came to Earth under the sponsorship of Mater St. Germain.

Who Is Master St. Germain?

Master St. Germain is the Lord of the Seventh Ray of Freedom and Transformation and the Violet Ray. He became the guardian of the Violet Transmuting Flame, also known as the Violet Fire and the Flame of Forgiveness, which offers people the gift of freedom to remove limiting or discordant conditions. St. Germain was a Master of the ancient wisdom and knowledge of the Matter spheres and previously walked the Earth plane. This Master had the wisdom, strength, and courage to bring the I AM instructions to the world. His great work with humanity has been profoundly important, and through it all he has developed much patience with the people on Earth.

Master St. Germain offers the Violet Fire to humanity as an antidote for the low-frequency energy that you wish to remove from your auric field. Master St. Germain took the responsibility of purifying the Earth and all upon it as his mission and service to Earth. The reason

St. Germain revealed the knowledge of the Violet Fire to Guy Ballard, founder of the "I AM" Movement, in the 1930s was so humans could balance their karma more rapidly through the evoking of the mercy, love, and compassion qualities of the Violet Flame.[1]

What Is the Violet Fire?

The Violet Fire, also known as the Violet Transmuting Flame and the Sacred Fire, is one of the most powerful vibrational frequencies and enters our field of vision as ultraviolet and violet. This frequency operates to open our crown chakra and connect us to Source. It does so by purifying our whole body, removing blockages, and then transforming the negative energy into Light. The Violet Flame is a current of energy that has been qualified to seize negativity and disharmony and transmute it into a higher-frequency vibration.[2]

The Violet Fire is the divine alchemy that resurrects and perfects energy. It draws energy into a form or condition that alters it into something from the higher octaves. This is accomplished through invocation, visualization through focusing, and intention, and the intelligence within the Violet Fire changes the vibratory action of a situation.[3]

The Violet Fire is a cosmic gift, a spiritual tool with which you can harmoniously transmute all wrong conditions and anything that is less than pure divinity. The Violet Fire erases negative karma permanently. If you use it sufficiently, you can erase from your life stream everything that is not of the Light that has ever accumulated in your energy system. It does not repress karma, but it changes the vibratory action and makes the discord non-existent. As you call for the Violet Fire, a ray comes from the hands, heart, and head of your I AM Presence, and as it touches the surface beneath your feet, it bursts into flame.[4]

Since violet is the seventh and highest frequency within the color spectrum of visible light, when projected into any situation or problem it manifests as an energy field of transmutation whereby alchemy or cosmic change may occur. The Violet Fire allows the dissolving of age-old records of karma because of the inherent qualities of Divine power (blue) and Divine love (pink), which, when merged, create a pulsating violet energy that consumes the darkness within all it touches.[5] The activity of the Violet Fire, once activated through the invocative power of thought, feeling, and the spoken word, is purification—it is a spiritual cleanser. It transmutes and returns back to the Universe anything that has fulfilled its service and is of no further use.[6]

In her book *The Next Step,* Patricia Cota-Robles states that the Violet Fire acts as an atomic accelerator and raises the frequency of chaotic energy in the environment into the vibrations of harmony. Throughout eons of time, humanity has created a world that is out of balance. The continual turmoil and stress in the emotions of individuals have created destructive conditions, problems, limitations, and struggles with the ego. This human creation can never be consumed or disposed of in any way, except by use of the Violet Fire.[7]

The Violet Flame, a neutralizing, controlling, and remolding activity of Divine love, consumes and transmutes wrong conditions and all that is less than perfect. It is a high rate of vibration that cleanses the force fields of electrons composing the atom, which produces a change in vibratory action and results in divine alchemy. You can call it forth into action in, through, and around you, as often as you wish. The Violet Fire's transmuting activity is as scientific and practical as melting ice (over a fire) into water, with greater heat turning it into steam. Through the use of Violet Fire, the vibratory action is changed, which changes the consistency of negative energy. The Violet Fire may be compared to a Good Cosmic Eraser. When used effectively, an individual can erase from his or her life all that is not of the Light that has accumulated in the cells of the body. Just imagine it working like a giant chalkboard eraser, wiping out feelings of pain, despair, suffering, and limitation, rubbing off and consuming the imperfection around the Points of Light in the body. Just like you erase a pencil mark on the paper, or clean a substance off the wall, you take off the dirty substance by your effort. The Violet Fire has exactly the same consuming activity in the cells of the body. Through the use of the Violet Fire, negative forces that are hindering you from success can be eliminated.[8]

In physicality, Violet Light has the highest frequency in the visible spectrum. This same vibratory frequency, combined with the element of fire, can consume discord within and between the atoms of our Being. The color of the Violet Flame ranges from pale lilac to magenta to deep amethyst, according to its intensity. Visualize the Violet Flame passing through your heart to remove fear and doubt, resentment, and lack of compassion. However, some issues may still necessitate processing via psychological therapy.[9]

How It Works

When you use the Violet Fire, it removes the impure substance from the brain structure and the feeling from your emotional body. This is the impure substance that can connect you to disturbing situations in the environment. Consequently, when you use the Violet Fire around an individual, the density disappears, and they are compelled to see the Light within—whether they want to or not.

When heavy human density is wedged in between the electrons that make up each atom, it causes the atoms to spin more slowly and not in rhythm with the flow of your life-force energy. The Violet Fire accelerates the vibrations of the electrons and atoms and restores them to their rightful purity, thus allowing them to release perfect Light rays.[10] Therefore, if your mental body is sluggish, it is so because the spaces between the electrons that make up the atoms are clogged, just as your pencil sharpener gets so filled with filings that it does not function well. When the spaces between the electrons are filled with the energy caused by depression, discouragement, resentment, and frustration, the mental body ultimately begins to vibrate more and more slowly, until it is so sluggish that it is no longer receptive to the higher octaves for thoughts and inspirations.[11]

The Violet Fire functions by transmuting negative energies, thereby changing the vibrations (known in physics as oscillations) of the electrons in our body. When the density within the atom is removed, the electrons whirl faster, hold more Light, and raise our vibrations. For personal use, visualize the Violet Fire and then imagine it pouring into your physical body and filling every cell. Then bring it through your emotional, mental, and etheric bodies separately.

To clean a space such as your office or home, imagine the Violet Fire rising from the floor, consuming all low-frequency energy. It is especially important to pay attention to cleaning your bed with the Violet Fire when you get up in the morning.[12]

The Violet Fire can transmute subconscious blocks and patterns of darkness that hinder your soul development. It first dissolves certain underlying momentums that you have held in the basement of consciousness for lifetimes. These limiting momentums are replaced with positive new Light patterns. In this way you can quickly move into higher realms of Divine consciousness on your spiritual path.

No matter what needs to be corrected, the moment you call the Violet Fire to enter into a condition to correct what is wrong, its first action is to *shut off any expansion of the wrong.* The Violet Fire sweeps into all astral and psychic opposition and human conditions in your world. The Violet Fire cannot hurt anybody or anything. It simply dissolves what is wrong. It harmonizes and balances everything. When the Flash of the Violet Fire goes through, it purifies the substance and calms the energy in the emotional body.[13]

The Violet Fire frees you from the limitations of this world, whether they are in your body, your mind, your relationships, your immediate environment, or the world around you. It harmonizes and balances everything, so you cannot overuse the Violet Fire. In fact, the more you use the Violet Fire, the more it will bless you. The more it becomes real and the more you draw it forth from others, the more you automatically raise your vibrations. Now is the time to bring Light to those still in the shadows who are unable to break free.

Activities and conditions such as those related to war, hatred, power, and greed have been created and generated by humanity and affect the mind as well as the feelings of human beings—their toxic accumulations have been deposited down through the ages. With the consistent use of the Violet Fire, the mass accumulation of the centuries can be annihilated.[14]

Since use of the Violet Fire, for the most part, is not seen by physical sight, very few recognize and feel its essence and reality. Those of you who have inner vision and/or are kinesthetic can discern the Violet Fire and often have felt the changing of the vibratory action of your own bodies, as well as the dissolution of shadows by the power of the Light, and the removal of chaotic conditions in yourself and others through its use.[15]

The use of the Violet Fire daily is imperative, as it has a cumulative effect. The rapid positive vibration accelerates the energies of the four lower bodies and helps repel feelings of depression, doubt, fear, and lethargy as it assists the body to release all energy that is out of balance.[16]

When To Use It

You can invoke the Violet Fire by your focused intention alone. Simply imagine or visualize the Violet Fire passing through your physical body. Then stand there a few moments feeling as deeply as you can its rushing presence through your body and around you for a radius of three feet in every direction. See all excess substance, chaos, stress, limitation, negativity, or conflict dissolve. Then imagine all density and all substance within the body that is not pure, free, and of the Light slowly passing out at the top of your head through the Violet Fire, just like dark puffs of smoke or a shadow.

In this manner you can also free Mother Earth from excess negative energy. First, visualize the Violet Fire in and around individuals, situations, and geographical locations. Next, whenever you think of the Earth, visualize it as if it is a Violet Sun in space and the humanity of Earth as Ascended Beings who are already free. Also, through intention, remove the entire psychic stratum in the atmosphere of Earth—this is a layer of energy within which particular vibrations are constantly acting, accumulating, and condensing into destructive activities at certain points in the atmosphere of Earth.[17]

The Violet Fire soothes the whirls of stress in the emotional body and consumes the substance that has caused the fear or doubt. Whether you think you need it or not, just call forth the Violet Fire whenever you feel irritated, disturbed, or uneasy. The Violet Fire comes to purify the substance and the energy in any situation. It is best to invoke the Violet Fire before you start your day. The Violet Fire needs to be used before you do anything in this world, day after day, many times a day. Then you stand insulated in your tri-colored bubbles of protection.

You might consider flooding everything that is on your schedule for the day with the Violet Fire for a few minutes before you start your day's activities; it can often clear your way of conditions in the world that are not of your creation but rather are part of the mass accumulation of humanity's past thoughts and feelings. Experiment with calling it into situations for just one day in everything you do. Just give it a Flash. In one day, see what it will do for you to make your path easier. It can calm your mind and feelings as it releases tension, strain, and struggle from your emotional body. You can even charge yourself the night before with the energy you're going to use the next day.[18]

Whenever there seems to be any disturbance, or when you're under stress, struggling, too tired, or just easily irritated, do not let that feeling build to the place where it exhausts you and drains your energy. Instead, call forth the Violet Fire to flood in and around you, to purify everything, and to remove the disturbing situation. This will always keep your intellect, the outer consciousness of the personal self, free from so many things that hold your attention and the thoughts that take your energy or keep your attention on something destructive. This will help you develop Mastery over the ever-changing conditions of the physical world.[19]

To work with the Violet Fire, call Master St. Germain to your I AM Presence, along with Archangel Zadkiel and the Angels of the Violet Flame. These Beings all work on the Seventh Ray (the Violet Ray) and work with the Violet Fire extensively. Ask them to help you use the Violet Fire.

Repeat the following Cosmic Law of Forgiveness a minimum of three times. Doing or saying things three or seven times with emphasis has ancient spiritual significance and is very powerful. There is a reason the decree includes a call for all humankind. Using the Violet Fire for all humankind is a great service to those who do not know that the Violet Fire exists. It is one way to serve others anonymously and help the planet move into Light. It is best to call on the Cosmic Law of Forgiveness just before calling for the Violet Fire. By calling for the many, you enable greater forgiveness for yourself.[20] Then say:

I call upon my I AM Presence or the Law of Forgiveness for myself and all humankind for all mistakes, misqualified energy, human consciousness, and the straying from the Light. I ask the Violet Fire to blaze through and around me and purify and transmute now all impure desires, hard feelings, wrong concepts, imperfect etheric records, causes, cores, effects, and memories, known or hidden. Keep this flame sustained and all-powerfully active. Replace all by pure substance, power of accomplishment, and the Divine plan fulfilled.

You can repeat the call several times (three or seven) in succession, at least in the beginning, as it helps to anchor and make it real in your consciousness. Meanwhile, picture (mentally see) the Violet Flame, like a soothing flame penetrating your Being and world, right up through your body, organs, bones, and all. The physical body is not completely solid, as it seems. Instead, it is composed of energy vibrating at various oscillations.

It is necessary to demand the removal of every picture that has ever registered in your consciousness that did not produce success for you, because within your memory—which is located in both your mental and your emotional bodies, and also your etheric body—the pictures are held that were the force to produce the manifestations of the past, be they good or otherwise.

These negative vibrations may get into a person's auric field from within accumulations of discord, which are recorded in the etheric body and that are sometimes brought to the surface by the outer consciousness. Negative vibrations may also get into the person's world because they float in the atmosphere in which the person moves. Finally, negative vibrations may enter a person's world because they may consciously be directed to him or her by others.[21]

How To Use It

Using Violet Fire in your everyday existence can be a fairly easy adaptation. Simply visualize a pillar of whirling violet consuming flame enfolding everyone, and extracting into itself everything that is of the impurity, and the distress and limitation of the outer self's creation. Visualize a flame as you might see it in the fireplace, but see it violet or purple in color. It is getting the feeling of it that truly brings results.[22]

If you find it difficult to hold your peaceful and balanced harmonious feeling in the aura of someone whom you may have allowed to disturb your feelings, you can call the Violet Fire silently while in their presence, for the instantaneous manifestation of Violet Fire to transmute that appearance of discord into loving feelings of peace and harmony.[23]

If you are troubled or irritated by someone in your immediate vicinity, call forth the Violet Fire and picture yourself (as well as the other person) within the center of the flame. It can assist you with the purification of your relationship. Furthermore, if there is a stressful or negative situation around you, or you have feelings you wish to cleanse, you can visualize the Violet Fire and mentally step within it.[24]

Try to feel as often as you can that when you have called or visualized the Violet Fire in Action, it is sustained there. Blaze the Spinning Flame around a condition, or blaze the flame through the situation as much as you can, and when you hold the picture within your mind as you call its action into conditions, try to feel that the flame is established there. Mentally see it burning like you keep a fire fed.

When you build a fire in your home to keep it warm, you keep it sustained; you keep feeding it. Well, when you ask the Violet Fire to be focused in the government, for example, or in and around individuals, as you hold the mental picture see it in continuous action. Whenever you think of it, always see it in the situation, and see the situation surrounded by the flame. When you think of an individual, see the Violet Fire blazing in and around him, as if his clothing were blazing with that Violet Fire, within and around. Then when you next think of the individual, think of the Violet Fire first, before you see the body within it.

If you will always give recognition to the existence of the Violet Fire, you strengthen it every time you think of the individual, because every time you hold the picture, you have intensified the flame's action. As an example, you can visualize the city you live in held within a Violet Sun of purifying energy. See the Violet Sun enter into the ground and see every person within the city blazing with the Violet Fire. Then call it to any other country.[25]

When you use the Violet Fire from the feet up, send it rushing up through the body and the atmosphere about you. It is the Purifying Love and Power that purges all the negativity. It is also the vibratory action in the atmosphere about you that sweeps out the discordant conditions in your feeling world. It consumes the substance thrown off by the negativity of others around you.[26]

The three-dimensional world is a continual flowing current of energy, substance, and vibration—destructive or otherwise. So as you recognize and use the Violet Fire in and around yourself, try not to think of it as just passing through or around you for a few moments—try to feel that it lives continually within you.

Alternatively, see the Violet Fire flash like a swirling tornado as it sweeps through a thing and then disappears. The vibratory frequency of the color and the action of the Violet Fire as it comes into you, goes into, and qualifies all the energy of your emotions will also flow through your brain structure. Since Violet Fire is wholly harmonious, you can only draw back into yourself that which will bless, purify, raise, and enhance you. You can request that your body rest within the Violet Fire and give you everything you need before you wake up. It will ease all your feelings by harmonizing them because it is very soothing. It will supply you with what you require. Charge yourself before you go to bed at night or even intermittently in the daytime.[27]

You can also hold the picture of those Pillars of Whirling Violet Fire enfolding everyone at your workplace, and drawing out and into itself everything that is of the impurity, and the distress, and limitations of the outer self's creation. You can flash it ahead of you like a River of Cosmic Light Substance for half an hour or an hour, or maybe on the instant. This is the technique I used on a daily basis during my half-hour commute to work when I lived in Ashland, Oregon. For three years I was a nurse manager in a rehabilitation facility in a neighboring town. During my daily ride to work on the freeway, I evoked the Violet Fire to travel ahead of me, clearing all negativity on the highway all the way to my work destination. Then I intended that the Violet Fire move through the entry of the facility, down the hall into my office to cleanse away all negative energy that may have accumulated in the area overnight. Next, while still driving, I evoked the full gathered momentum of the Violet Fire to move into each specific area of the building, including the dining room and each patient's room. When I finally did arrive at my job, I felt the energetic shift in the building and noticed that staff members and the patients were smiling easily.

When evoking the Violet Fire for yourself, imagine the flames blazing up, in, through, and around your four lower bodies (especially through your brain matter) as you command it to transmute any heavy and unforgiving thoughts and feelings in your etheric, mental, physical, and emotional bodies. These "hard" feelings, incidentally, are the causes and cores of most of your distresses. Then let these be replaced by grateful, receptive, joyful feelings.[28]

Currently, you have great opportunities to call forth this Violet Fire into this physical world, around persons, places, conditions, and things where it is most needed. To have the most efficacious use of the purifying activity of the Violet Fire, it is best to utilize it for short periods and not to stay at it too long. It is much more effective to call it forth more often, for shorter periods of time, in a rhythmic manner. Set aside some uninterrupted time each day, even if only five minutes at a time (say, three times a day, morning, noon, and night) to invoke the Violet Fire, calling it to blaze up, through, and around you. It is important to focus on the feeling of its activity in, through, and around you, then expand it outward into the world.[29]

Start at the feet and move upward. Hold the picture of everyone walking within the Violet Fire, as if you and they walked in water that was Violet Flame instead of water, up to a level just below the Heart. Command the energy three times a day in your emotional body first. It is a purifying and balancing force. Command, and ask it to blaze within, around, through you, and before you to clear away any and all negativity.[30]

In addition, you can use the Violet Fire during any healing sessions with Source. Your guides can help you to use the flame efficiently. When working with the Violet Fire, picture a soothing flame, as in a fireplace, only violet in color. See it penetrating you and your environment: all through your body and in the spaces between your cells. See it blazing through your emotional, mental, physical, and etheric bodies. You can say: *"Blaze the Violet Fire through my four lower bodies and keep this flame ever blazing."*

Then visualize it moving through these bodies. It is the feeling of the flame that brings the results that make you feel lighter. After your use of the flame, you have cleared out negativity in yourself. The space where you removed the negativity will remain clear unless you accumulate the same old negative stuff. You can consciously requalify it with constructive qualities by saying something like this: *"I ask my I AM Presence to charge me with perfect health, joy, happiness, illumination, love, wisdom, power, and abundance."*[31]

Violet Fire Decrees

1. Blaze, blaze, blaze the Violet Fire in, through, and around every part of my physical, mental, emotional, and etheric bodies, including my chakras. *(Repeat three times)*

   Remove and root out all the causes, cores, records, effects, and memories of misqualified energies stored within my chakras, right now and always. *(Repeat three times)*

   Restore the condition and shape of my chakras to their original perfection, as Source intended them to be. Beloved I AM. *(Repeat three times)*[32]

   I AM a force of Violet Fire more powerful than any human creation. *(Repeat three times)*[33]

2. Violet Fire, thou love divine,

   Blaze within this heart of mine!

   Thou art mercy forever true,

Keep me always in tune with you.[34]

I AM a Being of Violet Fire

As you say the following decree, visualize the Violet Flame bathing and cleansing all levels of your aura. Imagine all negative energy within, around, and through you being dissolved by the Violet Fire. You can use your creativity to create personalized variations of this theme.

1. *I AM a Being of Violet Fire!*
   I AM the purity Source desires!
2. *My family is a family of Violet Fire!*
   My family is the purity Source desires!
3. *My home is a home of Violet Fire!*
   My home is the purity Source desires!
4. (Name your state) *is a state of Violet Fire!*
   (Name your state) *is the purity Source desires!*
5. (Name your city) *is a city of Violet Fire!*
   (Name your city) *is the purity Source desires!*
6. (Name your country) *is the land of Violet Fire!*
   (Name your country) *is the purity Source desires!*
7. *Earth is a planet of Violet Fire!*
   Earth is the purity Source desires!

In addition to substituting your hometown, city, state, and country, you can use names of individuals instead of the I AM in the first decree.[35]

1. *My heart is a chakra of Violet Fire!*
   My heart is the purity Source desires![36]
2. *Expand, expand, and intensify daily the mightiest action of the Violet Fire in, through, and around my emotional, mental, etheric, and physical bodies, transmuting all negative energy into Divine love.*
3. *Expand, expand, and intensify daily the mightiest action of the Violet Fire in, through, and around all nationalities, races, and creeds in every country of the world, and in, through, and around the homes, places of employment,*

and general environment of all people until the Divine plan manifests for all life.

Become still and visualize how the destructive cause and cores embedded in your chakras are rooted out, one by one, similar to the action of removing a rubber suction cup.[37]

Daily Mantra to Ward Off Negative Vibrations

As previously stated, negative vibrations may enter a person's auric field as a result of his own accumulations of discordant thoughts, which are recorded in his etheric body and sometimes brought to the surface by outer consciousness. Negative vibrations may also enter a person's world because they float in the atmosphere in which the person moves, and/or negative vibrations may be consciously directed to him by others. In any case, the following decrees can be beneficial.[38]

You can invoke the Violet Flame by giving the following mantra. Try repeating it as you go about your day.

I AM a Being of Violet Fire!
I AM the purity God or Source desires!

Another powerful affirmation is to state, *"I AM the Violet Flame."* This connects your I AM Presence directly with the Violet Flame.[39]

Forgiveness

As stated earlier, the Violet Flame carries the energy of mercy, love, and forgiveness. The first step on the path toward Source is to forgive yourself and everyone else—all you have ever wronged and all who have wronged you. As you say the "Forgiveness" mantra, visualize spheres of Violet Flames going forth from your heart. See these spheres going to everyone you know, especially those with whom you've had struggles or strife. Visualize the Violet Fire going to that person and blessing him. Release all sense of injury or judgment into the Flame. The Violet Flame can consume the cause, effect, record, and memory of the wrong, re-establishing your heart in the oneness of love. Repeat the following mantra often and see how your life will change.

I AM forgiveness acting here.
Casting out all doubt and fear,
Setting people forever free
With wings of cosmic victory.

I AM calling in full power
For forgiveness every hour;
To all life in every place
I flood forth forgiving grace.

As you charge the pure light of Source with the Violet Flame, you can send out millions of Violet Flame spheres for the transmutation of the whole Earth. You *can* do something to change the world![40]

Violet Fire Meditations

Meditation for Fear, Anxiety, Depression

In order to become lighter and full of love, you must be willing to release your burdens, attachments, and limitations. Then forgiveness needs to be employed. The following meditation is an exercise for the emotional healing of fear, anxiety, and depression and is adapted from Pam and Fred Cameron's book *Bridge into Light*.[41]

Start your meditation with your usual routine. Center yourself and concentrate on your breathing. Visualize a sphere of golden white light around you as you call upon Master St. Germain. Then silently affirm, *"I AM one with the Violet Fire."* Repeat this to yourself several times until you feel aligned with that statement.

Now, visualize Violet Flames filling the entire room. You can imagine that from underneath the floor, etheric Violet Flames are moving into and surrounding the entire room. They extend up to the ceiling. Etheric energy is showering down in a gentle yet penetrating way to assist you in loosening up and releasing the clouds that have clung to your emotional body. The Violet Fire is the antidote to karma. You need not fulfill and live out your karma. You can call upon the Violet Fire and, by perseverance and acceptance, your karma can be resolved.[42]

Now, feel your body filled with the beautiful Violet Fire. Feel it growing and raising your vibration as it does. You have but to simply sit and breathe consciously. Pause and relax. If you feel your attention drawing you away, you can reaffirm that you are one with the Violet Fire. This will assist you in maximizing your experience.

Connect within yourself, within your emotions or feelings or thoughts, to a certain area of your life. Hold it within your hands and simply hold your hands out and visualize yourself releasing that area of your life into the intensification of the Violet Fire. Then declare out loud what you are releasing to the Universe.

The Violet Fire can assist you in raising the frequency of your vibrations and removing obstacles. It may seem subtle to you at first. Be assured that it works regardless of how powerfully you are able to experience each manifestation. Your sincere intention is everything.[43]

Whenever you set into motion the Violet Fire in and around yourself, or in outer-world conditions, ask your I AM presence to manifest in you whatever fulfills the Divine plan specifically of what you are calling forth. That will clear the way, and as a result things will manifest more rapidly for you.[44]

Violet Fire for Financial Abundance

Often people's cash-flow lines become blocked for a number of reasons. These blockages restrict the flow of financial abundance, rather than totally shutting it down. Some of the underlying causes of these personal cash-flow blockages are: attitudes of lack and limitation; vows of poverty taken in a previous lifetime; apathy toward financial goals; unresolved feelings of unworthiness; self-limiting messages through words, thoughts, and actions; and mental imprinting from parents regarding the value of money.

The following method to open cash-flow lines was created by the guidance I received:

I command that the Violet Transmuting Flame blaze, spin, and swirl within, around, and through my cash-flow lines (personal or business), blasting away any and all obstacles and blockages and transmuting all negativity into Divine love. I command that my cash-flow lines (personal or business) now be filled to capacity with God's Light, God's Grace, and God's Love that never fails, and my cash-flow lines now be surrounded by Violet Fire and guarded by the Blue Angels.

Optional:

I invoke the Three-Fold Flame. Blaze the blue light of Divine power through my cash-flow lines, the gold light of Divine wisdom through my cash-flow lines, and the pink light of Divine love through my cash-flow lines.

I command the Violet Transmuting Flame to blaze, spin, and swirl within, around, and through my four lower bodies and release any and all connections to lack, limitation, and poverty consciousness from this or any previous lifetimes. I renounce and rescind all vows of poverty that I have made in this or any other lifetime. I call upon the Angels of Protection to guide, protect, and overshadow me as I accept financial abundance as my true birthright. So Be It.

Chapter 7

Spiritual Power Tools

The following Spiritual Power Tools have been used throughout time to help members of humanity attune to their Higher Selves and Source. The specific Spiritual Power Tools that I was guided to mention in this chapter are techniques to enhance your spiritual empowerment as you journey on your path to ascension. The function of these specific spiritual tools is to alter your regular patterns of consciousness, so you can access your thoughts through different vibratory frequencies. Some of these power tools I will discuss are: visualizations, meditations, flower essences, Violet Fire, colors, chants, and decrees.

In some of the guided meditations in this book, you will be asked to imagine Light of different colors. It is important to trust that some part of your being knows how to create that Light and that particular color. As I stated before, "Intention is everything"!

Visualizations

Through the power of your mind you can create a new reality with imagination, contemplation, and intention. Specific visualization techniques are described that can increase the Light quotient in your body and release negativity. Implementing creative visualizations allows you to activate your inner senses, cleanse your energy fields, and further develop your higher mind.[1]

Sword of Blue Flame

This Sword is available to remove any whirls of discord in the emotional body that cause fear and doubt. With its electronic pattern it can in one flash do in an instant what it might take you much longer to feel in your use of the Violet Fire. The Violet Fire has the same power to consume doubt and fear instantly, but you do not always have the feeling within you of its immediate action, like you do with the Sword of Blue Flame. It strikes into everything discordant, to wipe it out from the world and the life stream to whom it was connected.[2]

In order to cut oneself free from destructive forces and connections of this incarnation and all former ones, the following applications can be used. First give attention and love to your I AM Presence and feel it envelop your hand and arm while you visualize a Sword of Blue Flame in your hand. Then with your physical hand go through the motion of cutting down all around you with the sword, turning your body around until the circle is completed, severing all ties and strings connecting you with forces of fear, doubt, and others outside yourself (which may be anywhere on Earth or in its atmosphere). Then ask your I AM Presence to blaze forth light rays to the furthest ends of the lines of force connected with you and return them all the way back to you, transmuting whatever is not of the Light. In this way one can get rid of a lot of imperfect karma in a short time.[3]

When we move into action with the Sword of Blue Flame and the Circle of Blue Flame (see page 109), it removes the destructive etheric record that is the focus of its action—this "record" is accumulated energy by which it can produce destructive activities in a person's life. Archangel Michael releases at your call in, through, and around whatever negative energy you designate in that call.[4] This sword can cut through whatever destructive condensations of energy you designate when you call it forth to shatter and transmute those negative energies.[5] In addition to the severing and uprooting of negative forces described above, the Sword of Blue Flame may be called upon for strength, power, and protection.

Circle of Blue Flame

The Blue Flame is greatly concentrated powerful energy that must always be used with love.[6] It is a ring of spiritual blue-white fire that may be invoked to immobilize negative situations. This circle can surround you up to ten feet in all directions. Visualize this around your solar plexus, around the middle of the body (like a belt), with your definite command that it shall never vibrate to any negativity. This protective Circle of Blue Flame will repel and consume suggestions directed at your emotional body before they can connect with you. Then imagine the Circle of Blue Flame closing in completely around the center of the body. This will be an armor of protection for the energy of your emotional body. It will conserve your strength and improve your health. Psychic suggestion and other forces of the psychic stratum in the atmosphere of Earth reach you more easily through the emotional body than they do by suggestion to the mind. Be aware of this possibility at least three times a day and particularly at times when your feelings are excited, disturbed, resentful, or negative in any way. Immediately focus on this Circle of Blue Flame around you.

When invoked, the Circle of Blue Flame forms around a situation in order to prevent the negativity from spreading. It is often used together with the Sword of Blue Flame to cut individuals free from negative astral interferences. You can see or imagine this spiritual tool surrounding an individual at the waist, or around entire groups of people, buildings, entire cities, states, countries, and around the Earth at the equator as it releases layers of density.

As stated previously in Chapter 5, "Spiritual Protection," this is an added protection that surrounds the Pillar of Light. Just ask your I AM Presence to surround your Pillar of Light with the Circle of Blue Flame and also to give you any added protection that is required. Then state your gratitude. Next, picture this Circle of Blue Flame completely surrounding your Pillar of White Light. See it about four inches thick.[7]

In the name of my beloved I AM Presence, I invoke an invincible shaft of Blue Flame to be placed over me. Let it surround every cell, atom, and electron of my Being. Let this shaft of Sapphire Blue Light expand into my various bodies and all my chakras.

Cut me free from everything that is less than the highest light within me. Let the Blue Flame of Divine love guard my force field of protection, daily and hourly. I know that I AM absolutely protected at all times and in all places. I express my deep gratitude for all assistance given unto me always. Amen.[8]

Wall of Blue Flame

This spiritual tool enters into a situation to consume what is negative and to shut off its expansion. Drop it around the situation and encircle it, until it is immovable and the Flame consumes it.[9] When you use the Wall of Blue Flame for protection around all that is constructive, it becomes the "Cloak of Invisibility," but it also becomes a sustaining energy to whatever it is protecting.

The Cross of Blue Flame

Imagine a Cross of Blue Flame in front of all the entrances to your home to cleanse negativity from all who enter. Call this forth when you feel you need protection, and also to silence and hold inactive destructive forces.[10]

The Spiral Blue Flame

This can be used to encircle destructive forces, cores, and causes and to extract and transmute them.[11]

The Cosmic Blue Lightning

This is concentrated energy of the fire element. It is an action of Divine love and is used to purify the dense substance, especially wherever there is hatred, intolerance, and selfishness. The use of the Cosmic Blue Lightning of Divine love and purity is the only way or means to purify some of the density of Earth substance. It is likened to a bolt of electricity capable of shattering all illusion. It has a consuming and transmuting power, but its main action is to shatter into pieces any masses of negative or destructive energy. It goes into the destructive center and shatters apart the vortex, the central focus that has created and expanded the accumulation. It not only consumes the immediate human accumulation, it consumes the destructive etheric record. (The etheric records are a collective of the past history of everything that has transpired in the physical world. These records exist on a higher plane that holds all the memories of our souls.) Then such an accumulation can be more easily and quickly transmuted by the Violet Fire.[12] There are also Legions of Angels of Blue Lightning that can be called forth to assist you when needed.[13]

Then, after the Blue Lightning passes through and shatters apart the accumulated substance, the Violet Fire can be called forth for the final Purification.

Mantras

Throughout time, mantras, decrees, and chants have been used by a wide variety of religions to attune to the Higher Self.[14] Some people don't realize that a mantra or decree is actually a force field of energy that is reinforced each time it is given. This is why the Our Father and the Hail Mary are so powerful—because they have been given by devotees again and again for centuries.

A mantra is a word or phrase (often with spiritual significance) repeated over and over while meditating or doing other spiritual practices. The repetition of the name or sound serves to keep you focused during the meditation and is often uplifting as well. The vibration of the sacred tones can shift the energy in a person or a place. The mantra can also function as a focusing mechanism for the mind to produce calmness and clarity. "As without, so within" means that if our minds are not clear, we are prone to creating the external turbulence in our environment. The following mantras can be utilized to create peace and harmony in your home setting as well as your mind. This will be realized over time as you commit to the regular utterance of the chants, as it takes a period of time for a mantra to become fully effective. The great peace mantra is *OM SHANTI, SHANTI, SHANTI* and is for personal and global peace. This is translated as *Om Peace! Peace! Peace!*[15]

Mantras and chants are spiritual tools that can help us attune to our higher selves and our pure state of spiritual being. Throughout the ages in a wide variety of religious and spiritual practices, mantras or chants have been used in order to gain the desired effect. The most familiar mantra of the East is the chanting of the sound *Om* or *Aum*.[16]

Another widely used mantra of the East is the Buddhist chant of *Om-Mani-Padme-Hum*. It is from Tibet and translates as "Hail the Jewel in the Lotus." The jewel in this case is the Buddha of Compassion.[17]

Another powerful mantra is based on the Holy Name of Shiva, the Hindu destroyer of negativity. This mantra, *Om Namah Shivaya,* is believed to prepare us for personal renewal and transformation. Liberation from outmoded concepts and beliefs helps us be ready to accept new challenges and embrace fresh opportunities.[18]

Tube of Light Mantra

Beloved I AM Presence bright,
Round me seal your Tube of Light
From Ascended Master flame
Called forth now in God's own name.
Let it keep my Being free
From all discord sent to me.

I AM calling forth Violet Fire
To blaze and transmute all desire,
Keeping on in freedom's name
Till I AM one with the Violet Flame.[19]

Decrees

A decree is a fiat, a command to invoke the presence of God, his consciousness, his power and protection, purity and perfection.[20] Decrees can be given silently, but they must be imbued with feeling and conviction.

As the decrees go forth in a fairly rapid but balanced tempo, the rate of the vibration of the atoms making up your physical, etheric, emotional, and mental bodies increases to transmute discordant energies.[21]

The basis of any decree pattern is repetition. The decrees function as a balance for the misuse of the spoken word over centuries and for negative thought patterns created by humanity. In order to shatter these thought-forms, it is necessary to use energy vibrating at the same rate— but constructively positive. In other words, a thought pattern created by wrong speech must be broken by a vibratory action of correct speech. This concept is based on the fact that we have misused in many prior lifetimes much energy through the spoken word, and charged that into the mental, emotional, and etheric bodies. Consequently we have instilled qualities of negativity within them. In order to shift this negativity, we have to release a type of higher energy that will shatter these previous patterns created through the use of the spoken word.[22]

Through decrees you can contribute energy from the physical realm that is taken up and assimilated for the specified purpose. One-third of the energy must be released from human beings in the physical realm by intention; two-thirds of the energy will be supplied by the Universe. The real implementation of the power of the decree is not just saying words in the form of multiple decrees: one must feel the emotion and intent behind the words, or that energy will accumulate into more thought-forms that some day must be transmuted. We must watch that we do not get into a state of consciousness just making calls for release of energy; rather, we want to make the call for action. Decreeing takes one up to a certain point, but then it's necessary to do more than that—one needs to follow through. Empty decrees are a matter of energy released from the human side without enough love; the required follow-through is in making the call, holding the picture, and feeling enough love to activate the flame in the heart that gives the response from the Presence.[23]

By hearing a decree repeated three times, we become more and more convinced of the Truth we are phrasing aloud. That is why decrees that are voiced by a group are so very powerful. The need to repeat decrees when we have asked for them to be sustained is because we do not sustain them in our consciousness, especially our feelings. The reason we don't sustain the radiation from the Masters is that the substance from the outer world moves in on us again. After giving a decree you can say to your I AM Presence: "Keep it sustained and expanding."[24] After you recite the decree, rest within your I AM Presence. Visualize or imagine being totally enfolded in this great spiritual energy.

If you have negative energy and wish to hold on to it, decrees will not be effective since angels do not interfere with your free will. They will not release anger of any level unless you have made a decision to surrender it. The angel that comes to help you with unresolved feelings can only take what you are willing to relinquish. The following prayer can assist you in releasing any toxic emotions.

> *Dear Angels, Please help me to surrender this anger* [or name another emotion]. *Please send into my heart the Violet Transmuting Flame of mercy and forgiveness. Let it consume all hardness of my heart and any non-forgiveness of myself or others. Then replace it with love and compassion. So Be It; So Be It; So Be it! Amen.*[25]

Archangel Michael Decrees

The following are two decrees to Archangel Michael (repeat them three times):

Archangel Michael, Archangel Michael, Archangel Michael, I call unto thee:

Wield thy sword of blue flame
And now cut me free.

For traveling protection:

Archangel Michael before me, Archangel Michael behind me,
Archangel Michael to the right of me, Archangel Michael to the left of me,
Archangel Michael above, Archangel Michael below,
Archangel Michael, Archangel Michael, Archangel Michael, wherever I go!

The decree above for safe travel can be issued for your family, friends, and co-workers, as well as for the whole world.[26]

Flower Essences

Flower essences are designed to combat specific emotional and spiritual conditions such as fear, guilt, resentment, or a sense of inadequacy. These remedies assist with the cleansing of accumulations of emotions, healing patterns of reaction that accompany them, and increasing conscious awareness of more effective ways to cope with these emotions. They primarily work on our characteristics, attitude, and behavior.

Flower essences are created from the flowers of plants, bushes, and trees. The flower is picked when it is mature and preserved in mineral water. The energy of the plant with its unique qualities is then available for treating personality and many fixed emotional patterns that are difficult to eradicate by talk therapy alone. The different vibrational frequencies emitted by plants have been found to have varying effects on our emotional, spiritual, and mental bodies. The modern groundbreaker in this form of therapy was Edward Bach, who developed a holistic approach to health, disease, and healing through a range of flower essences that are now widely available. Bach Flower Remedies are wonderful tools for healing emotions on a subtle energy level. They can be purchased at health food stores, which usually also carry books describing their use.[27] There are thirty-eight different Bach Flower Remedies for balancing and correcting many emotional states, based entirely on negative soul states.[28]

Other essences have been developed using plants from different parts of the world, and you are probably best advised to use your local products, as they will suit local conditions. If you can't decide which remedy suits your personal requirements, then close your eyes and hold your hands over the selection and let your senses lead you to the one you need. The following remedies are especially helpful for lifting you out of negative thinking:

- Elm for being overwhelmed with responsibility
- Cerato for developing intuition

- Gentian for despondency
- Chicory for letting go of what you have been holding on to
- Gorse for hopelessness and despair
- Honeysuckle for being stuck in the past and not living in the present
- Mustard for sadness and feeling miserable for no obvious reason
- Oak for strength and endurance
- Olive for physical and mental fatigue
- Rock Rose for releasing anxiety and fear
- White Chestnut for a balanced state of mind
- Wild Rose for apathy[29]

Over the years I've used flower essences as a healing modality. My favorites come from a company called Perelandra. I've had excellent success with the Rose II Essences for both heart palpitations and ocular migraines. Their Soul Ray Essences are specifically designed to help the body assimilate and integrate soul-expansion experiences. For ongoing relief from stress, anxiety, and overwhelm, I find Bach Flower Rescue Remedy helpful, even for my grandchildren.

Aromatherapy

With the stresses and strains of life's pressures, we often become unbalanced. We lose sight of opportunities to allow our minds and bodies to recapture harmony. This imbalance occurs on a gradual basis and beneath our awareness. The residuals are reflected in our thoughts, attitudes, and actions. We often become so absorbed in our goals and material desires that we ignore the present moment and all that it holds for us. By using the essential oils of aromatherapy—aromatic liquids distilled from different flowers, plants, and herbs—you can assist your body and mind with regaining the forgotten equilibrium.

For centuries, essential oils have withstood the test of time for healing, combating infections, promoting relaxation, and uplifting the spirit.

Their unique chemical structure seems to promote healing by stimulating and strengthening the body's natural mechanisms through the powerful emotional sense of smell. Contemporary science has documented that a mere whiff of a fragrance can activate a series of reactions in our bodies that can affect us emotionally and energetically. Certain aromas may stimulate the release of body substances that can relax us, help focus our attention, or enhance our mood.

Aromatherapy is a fantastic modality because it utilizes the sense of smell. When essential oils are inhaled or diffused, the health benefits unique to each fragrance are released through the olfactory system (the biological mechanism of smell). The aromatic molecules of the essential oils absorb into the bloodstream from the nose to the limbic system that activates the amygdala (the memory center for pleasure).[30] This broad and expanding field of aromatherapy, recently rediscovered, is a gift from the past that you can use to improve the present day. The aromas of essential oils can soothe your mind, raise your energy level, heighten spiritual awareness, and promote restful sleep. Essential oils can be dropped in the bath, used directly on areas of concern, placed in an aromatic diffuser, mixed with massage oils, or inhaled directly.

I have been studying the health benefits of essential oils since I became enamored by them more than twenty years ago. In 1999, I created a series of aromatherapy spray mists from precise formulas that I received through my automatic writing during my meditations. These spray mists are sold online from my business called Healing Vibrations. The following oils will uplift spirits, energize, and help relieve depression:

- Bergamot has antidepressant qualities, relieves stress, and promotes creativity and a sense of well-being.
- Clary Sage assists with stress by reducing nervousness.
- Geranium has antidepressant qualities and promotes happiness.
- Lemon also has antidepressant qualities.
- Neroli, Nutmeg, Peppermint, and Spearmint assist with emotional rejuvenation.
- Basil, Rosemary, and Amber can increase mental clarity.

- Orange is mood-elevating and helps relieve nervous anxiety.
- Patchouli helps with stress-related situations by calming the nervous system.
- Grapefruit, Orange, Rose, and Frankincense help to balance depression.
- Ginger, Clove, Juniper, and Cinnamon help to alleviate mental fatigue.
- Rosewood is uplifting, energizing, and has antidepressant qualities.
- Jasmine has uplifting capabilities, helps revitalize energy, and increases vibrations.
- Ylang Ylang helps with depression, stress, and tension.[31]

Lavender has long been known for its relaxing effects. You can rub Lavender oil on your feet or behind your ears for a calming effect on your whole body. You also might consider rubbing a drop of Lavender oil on your palms and then smoothing it on your forehead or your pillow to help you sleep.

Peppermint is one of the oldest herbs for soothing digestion. Try rubbing a few drops of Peppermint essential oil in your palm and then around your navel area to relieve nausea or indigestion. To relieve a headache, rub a drop of Peppermint oil on your temples, forehead, and behind your ears. Peppermint oil also promotes concentration and stimulates thinking. I use it, or basil, in my car when I am driving a long distance.

Frankincense enhances one's connection to Spirit and fosters the development of intuition and inner guidance. It promotes a deep stillness and soothes, calms, and balances the mind and emotions. It is helpful in alleviating stress, tension, anxiety, and any other nervous disorders linked with a negative past or fear of the future.

The following Frankincense Meditation was shared with me over a decade ago by Randyl Rupar, PhD, from Hawaiian Wellness at the Sanctuary of Mana Ke'a.[32] According to Dr. Rupar, Frankincense works with the cellular memory of your body and helps you remember what you came here to do.

Frankincense Meditation and Anointing

(Opens crown, heart, and root chakras)

- Begin by setting your intention to link your body, mind, and spirit. Then place a drop of essential oil on your crown chakra and another one on the palms of your hands.
- Call forth the Angels of 100% pure Light.
- Place a few drops of Frankincense on your middle finger and forefinger and then draw an infinity symbol on your forehead.
- Draw a spiral on each temple. (This links the left and right hemisphere in harmony with each other so they will have the same brain wave frequency.)
- Place a drop of Frankincense under your nose, above your upper lip.
- Place a drop on your thymus gland to connect with your immune system.
- Rub your hands together to create heat in your palms and place your forefingers on the third eye and your thumbs on your temples.
- With your tongue on the roof of the mouth, breathe deeply three times.
- Affirm aloud three times that Peace, Love, and Joy fill your entire Being.
- Breathe in Love, Peace, and Joy separately and exhale each using nasal breaths.
- Place hands in prayer position and express your gratitude to the Universe.

The Infinity Symbol

Symbols can be powerful and time-honored representations. For example, the Infinity symbol is an abstract concept describing something without limits, and thus impossible to measure. In ancient India and Tibet, it symbolized perfection, dualism, and unity of male and female.[33] This symbol for eternity is the horizontal eight and represents one of the fundamental movements of atoms and molecules. As you work with the Infinity symbol, it seems to be exerting its influence on a subconscious level. You can accelerate this connection by choosing to use it in your daily life whenever possible. This symbol may be used physically as you trace the sideways figure eight with your hands or head. It may also be used with your inner vision as you trace the symbol repetitively.

One way you can utilize this symbol in gold and white is to imagine that it flows within, around, and through you in a swirling manner, as you connect with your angels, guides, and teachers of 100% pure Light. You can also swirl the Infinity symbol with your salad dressing over your foods, with olive oil when you cook, or with bath oil/gel as you draw your bath. As you walk out in nature, you can connect with the trees, flowers, or Mother Earth by imagining this very powerful symbol of oneness, filled with love and gratitude, flowing from you to each object and then back through your Being.

As you use the Infinity symbol on a regular basis, you will be subconsciously connecting with Source. This will increase your spiritual connection with "All That Is." Remember that your focus and intention are key. Then watch to see how this simple but powerful intention leads you to higher dimensions of consciousness.

In meditation you can imagine (or intend) that a pulsating Ray of White Light enters your crown chakra and begins to pass back and forth between the right and left hemispheres of your brain. As it does, it gently forms an Infinity symbol that then flows through all the pathways and meridians of your brain as it reconnects the circuits and heals all fragmented connections. This activity of the Infinity symbol balances the hemispheres of the brain and brings into equilibrium the masculine and feminine aspects of Divinity within your soul. Then the Ray of White Light travels down the front and back of your body into Mother Earth.

Infinity Symbol Exercise

This exercise can be done in either a sitting or standing position. It was adapted from one that Chris Griscom created years ago.[34] In your mind's eye you will be connecting your physical body with your I AM Presence with a figure-eight movement of Light.

- Make yourself comfortable, closing your eyes and allowing yourself to relax.

- Begin by taking in three deep breaths through your nose and then exhaling each through your mouth.

- Now imagine a soft crystalline pulsating ball of White Light at the base of your spine. Follow it as it becomes a stream of Light and travels up your spine, then up your neck until it reaches the top of your head at the crown area.

- Imagine that this pathway of Light energy extends over your head and twists at the level of your Higher Self, to make an arc as it moves upward over your I AM Presence. Notice, at this point, that half of the vertical figure-eight shape has been created.

- Now follow this stream of Light energy as it loops around your I AM Presence and moves back down, descending from the I AM Presence down to Higher Self, then down to the crown chakra toward your Higher Self as it twists again, crossing over its original path, on its way back toward your physical body.

- Follow the Light energy shaft now as it returns to your crown, cascades over your forehead and down the front of your body, between your legs, until it reaches the base of your spine again.

- The Infinity sign is now completed by linking your physical body with your I AM Presence.

- Visualize rainbow-colored energies arising from the Earth to the base of your spine. These rainbow-colored energies now follow the same route as the stream of Light, through your Higher Self to your I AM Presence. These energies then return to the base of your spine once again.

While implementing this exercise, you can let this Light energy flow at whatever pace is comfortable for you. At times this may result in a subtle vibrating or warmth sensation within or around your physical body. Often people will experience feeling more energized, balanced, and clear afterward.

Spiritual Stone Power

All things are of Source Energy, and everything that physically exists has a vibratory rate. The mineral kingdom manifests the lowest vibratory rate on the third-dimensional Earth plane. Consequently, the mineral kingdom is the foundation of all things on the physical plane—it is what they are made of, whether it is vegetable, animal, or human in nature (as you might remember from your science classes).

The most common elements of all living things are carbon, hydrogen, and oxygen. Even the human body is composed of organic and inorganic elements including carbon, hydrogen, nitrogen, oxygen, calcium, and phosphorus.[35]

Gemstones from the mineral kingdom are concentrated points of Light within the color spectrum. When they were brought forth from deep within the earth, it was discovered that they are not only beautiful, they possess powerful healing energies. Their healing qualities have long been known to humanity. In ancient civilizations their usage to eliminate physical disorders was developed into an exact science. With the dawn of Christianity, the healing benefits of gemstones were suppressed. This knowledge has now resurfaced in order to benefit those who are aligned with these earth energies. Each mineral crystal has its special individual influence, function, and vibration. Inherent in the evolution of the mineral kingdom are the vibratory rates that heal, energize, attune, and uplift the spirit of our inner Beings. The energy patterns of gemstones serve humanity in many ways. Some frequencies are conducive to meditation, inspiration, and reflection, while others affect our body's physical health.

As you progress along your spiritual path, there might be times when you find yourself in need of a certain missing vibration that would assist your growth. At these times you might be guided by your Higher Self, consciously or unconsciously, to seek some form of additional vibration, which often can be obtained from a gemstone or a mineral.[36] Many people choose to have a gemstone in their possession on a daily basis, to either wear or carry in their pocket or bra. In most cases, there is an intuitive need for that particular gemstone's vibrational additive. Another way you can experience guidance is when selecting a small quartz crystal or gemstone from a group or several. Frequently by just hovering the palm of your hand over a group of stones you can be drawn energetically to a certain one. While handling one, you may notice that it "feels" right to you.[37]

A variety of gemstones, not only quartz, can be used in several beneficial ways. Worn upon the physical body, a gemstone's unique electromagnetic force will strengthen the etheric body, at the same time it stimulates the physical form at the site it is worn. Those who suffer from disorders in the throat or general weariness due to worry or fear should consider the benefits of wearing a gem around the throat, particularly amber. Where there is tension in the region of the solar plexus due to increasing levels of sensitivity, a slice of polished agate or amethyst can help to deflect negative or destructive vibrations. If under psychic attack, a large piece of carnelian worn in the umbilical region is believed to be of great protective benefit.[38]

The natural, uncut stones often possess a far greater energy than those that have been cut and polished. Also, these are not as highly priced as those of gemstone quality. Once your favorite rough stones are selected, cleanse them by immersing them in sea salt and water for twenty-four hours to remove all residue. Then rinse them under cold water and they are immediately ready to be of service to you.

The following compilation-listing is not to be used to prescribe or diagnose in any manner. It is not a substitute for professional help. The intent is to offer historical and spiritual uses of stones and crystals in order to assist you in your spiritual development.[39]

Agate: Soothes the emotions
Integrates throat, heart, and solar plexus chakras
Imparts a sense of strength and courage
Grounding, but energetic; often used as a worry-stone
Increases inner awareness

Amazonite: Soothes the nervous system; aids alignment of mental and etheric bodies

Regulates thinking faculties

Self-expression; calming and soothing

Builds inner confidence and serenity; creativity

Helps you to see your surroundings with insight

Amber: Grounds and stabilizes; enhances patience

Draws out negative energy from the body

Mental clarity; lifts depression

Clears the mind and eases stress

Cleanses the environment of negative vibrations
Aligns mental and emotional bodies

Provides positive mental states, encourages peacefulness

Amethyst: Facilitates healing on spiritual, mental, emotional, and physical levels

Increases spiritual awareness and enhances psychic ability

Expands energy field; cleanser and spiritual stimulant

Frequently used in meditation

Promotes inner peace

Prevents depression; calming

Enhances right-brain activity and pineal and pituitary glands

Clarifies thinking and communication

Opens spiritual and psychic centers

Aquamarine: Raises vibrational level of the aura

Puts self in touch with higher mind; uplifting

Calming, soothing; reduces fear

Excellent meditation stone; corrects imbalances

Aids spiritual visions; brings serenity and peace

Enables one to express oneself creatively

Enhances clarity of mind

Physical/emotional/mental balancer; self-awareness

Helps you "go with the flow"

Aventurine: Attracts abundance; soothes emotions

Alleviates anxiety and eases fears

Courage in social and group situations

Purifies mental, emotional, and etheric bodies

Brings one into alignment with one's center

Promotes independence and originality

Helps to see alternatives and potentials; enhances creativity

Azurite: Used to release repressed emotions and for physical detoxing

Clarifies dreams; reduces depression

Enhances psychic abilities; cleanses the mental body

Stimulates thought; relaxes and rejuvenates

Facilitates clear meditation; opens to new awarenesses

Unites the subconscious with the consciousness mind

Strengthens the immune system; creativity; decisiveness

Develops self-confidence

Stimulates visual images during meditation

Bloodstone: Builds courage; invokes peace for the wearer

Helps in making decisions

Attracts good luck; reduces emotional/mental stress

Brings harmony to one's vibrations; enhances creative efforts

Aids self-confidence; adaptability; grounding

Stimulates flow of energy for all healing

Enhances physical/mental vitality; heightens senses

Removes emotional and physical blockages

Boji Stone: Aligns chakras; clears and charges aura; removes blockages

General healing and balancing; heals holes in the aura; mood elevator

Balances body's energy field; recharges electrically in the sun

Excellent to keep you centered in crowds; grounding

Calcite: Improves memory and intellect; energy amplifier

Balances male and female polarities

Strengthener in times of mental anguish

Assists in the transition to new ideas

Carnelian: Protects from negative thoughts; removes lethargy

Promotes inner peace; facilitates concentration

Aligns physical and etheric bodies

Dispels apathy; balances out the first chakra

Excellent for eliminating fear; enhances creativity

Instills confidence for public speaking

Helps awareness of feelings

Gives feeling of well-being; helps self-esteem

Celestite: Tunes to the higher mind; reduces stress

Used in meditation; aids personal creative expression

Fosters spiritual development

Disperses worries, brings balance, aids angelic communication

Promotes stillness for receiving

Enhances honesty

Charoite: Transmutes negativity, opens and balances the crown chakra

Relieves stress and overcomes fears; cleanses the aura

Good to use in meditation; stimulates inner vision

Helps to adjust to higher-frequency energy

Clears negative past-life patterning

Aids forgiveness of others; stone of transformation

Chrysocolla: Develops kindness, compassion, tolerance, and self-forgiveness

Helps clear subconscious imbalances

Develops inner peace; amplifies creative expression

Balances female endocrines

Eases nervous tension; increases psychic energy

Helps alleviate personal fears and guilt; draws prosperity

Aids the ability to speak one's truth

Eases the pain of anger or sorrow; meditation aid

Patience; cleanses auric field

Chrysoprase: Works on solar plexus and heart areas to soothe emotions

Used to absorb or deflect unwanted energies

Enhances insight into personal problems; uplifts

Aids tranquility; eases depression; makes one adaptable

Balances neurotic patterns; radiates peace and harmony

Healing for physical/emotional/mental bodies

Self-acceptance; self-confidence

Breaks up energy blockages

Citrine: Strengthens willpower

Heals the solar plexus

Draws prosperity

Stimulates healing of the physical body

Balances sexual energy; raises self-esteem

Generates radiant, happy vibrations

Opens the conscious mind to intuition; energizer

Promotes mental clarity

Enhances creativity

Coral: Strengthens nervous system, heart, and lungs

Protects from negativity; calms inner fears

Overcomes feelings of self-dislike; fosters compassion

Eases melancholy and excessive worry

Keeps thoughts in control for visualization and meditation

Emerald: Enhances memory; quiets emotions; promotes love

Balances will and wisdom; aids alignment of subtle bodies

Strong emotional balancer; draws prosperity

Helps one feel more positive; inspires deep knowing from within

Enhances mental powers; peaceful dreams

Promotes peace, harmony, and patience; lifts depression

Fluorite: Stimulates and opens the solar plexus; fosters truth

Unblocks energy flows; stress relief; uplifting

Grounds excess energy; opens creativity

Increases ability to concentrate

Good for meditation over third eye

Offers psychic protection and healing

Alleviates anxiety and hyperkinetic behavior

Strengthens ability to perceive higher levels of thought

Good for absorbing negative energies from the emotional body

Tetrahedron cleanses the aura in 30 seconds when held to third eye

Garnet: Enhances creativity; keeps energies flowing

Stimulates blood flow; aligns subtle bodies

Helps release fear; gives more energy

Helps alleviate depression; gives self-confidence and inspiration

Very grounding; has strong affinity with the root chakra

Aids in remembering dreams; stimulates happiness and fun

Helps us become more productive and achievement-oriented

Hematite: Grounding and centering influence to focus on the physical plane

Increases resistance to stress; enhances focus and concentration

Alleviates worry and anxiety as it allows for mental clarity

Increases physical vitality and improves self-esteem

Alleviates spaciness and increases intuition

Balances body, mind, and spirit; dissolves negativity

Strengthens physical and etheric bodies

Herkimer: Very balancing special variety of quartz crystal

Diamond: Works with yin-yang energies; promotes psychic abilities

Very highly attuned spiritually; clears static from aura

Stimulates visualization in meditation and dream work

Cleanses subtle bodies; energizing

Promotes dream recall and creativity; dissipates tension

Howlite: Calms, soothes, opens the mind; good for sixth and seventh chakras

Good with meditation; brings greater gentleness, patience

Fosters appreciation of beauty, inspiration, creativity

Artistic expression

Jade: Peaceful and nurturing; protection; self-confidence

Longevity, prosperity, and wisdom; grounding

Inspires quick and precise decisions; humility; practicality

Balances and soothes; dispels negativity

Brings good fortune to its owner; emotional balance

Does not absorb negative attributes of any nature

Helps us understand dreams and meditation

Jasper:

Energizes solar plexus and lower chakras

Strengthens one's will to do good; grounding

Balances the emotions; repairs aura tears

Helps people who need more organizational abilities

Relaxation, compassion, contentment

Kunzite:

Very high spiritual Love vibrations; confidence

Awakens and opens highest Heart consciousness

Great balance of compassion, peace, and freedom from fear

Balances emotional and mental bodies

Enhances self-esteem

Reduces depression

Clears the mental and emotional aspects of one's self

Kyanite:

Helps balance all chakras; enhances creative expression

Dispels frustration and anger; strengthens throat chakra

Good for meditating; aids in past-life regression

Enhances psychic images; tranquility

Assists with third-eye awakening; foresight

Encourages vivid dreams and clear visualizations

Lapis Lazuli:

Releases tension and anxiety; helps link to Higher Guidance

Enhances psychic abilities

Creative expression; energizes throat chakra; dream insight

Assists in opening and clarifying inner vision; meditation

Provides strength, vitality, and self-assurance; promotes truth

Stimulates mental clarity; intuition

Protection from psychic attack or negative thought-forms

Malachite: Strengthens and cleans auric field; draws prosperity

Clears solar plexus blocks; excellent for patience and self-control

Centers and protects; reduces stress and tension

Stimulates healing properties; absorbs negativity
Balance; concentration; inner clarity; self-understanding

Promotes subconscious understanding

Moonstone: Relieves anxiety and stress

Helps define and balance feminine energy

Stimulates intuition; fosters happiness

Enhances clairvoyance; good for meditation; stimulates pineal gland

Relieves frustration and balances emotions

Spiritual guidance and protection while traveling; spiritual insight

Obsidian: Used to sharpen both the internal and external vision

Stabilizes erratic energies; reduces stress; uplifts

Grounds and deflects negative energy

Absorbs negative energies from the environment

Introspection; psychic ability; dissolves anger and fear

Helps clear subconscious blocks

Onyx: Develops a sense of purpose, self-discipline, and foresight

Relieves stress and apathy; aids detachment; grounding

Manifests objective thinking; helps control negative thinking

Balances male/female polarities; relieves grief

Enhances self-control, especially for making wise decisions

Absorbs negativity; valuable in difficult or confusing times

Opal:
Bridges the lower mind with the Higher Self

Helps develop psychic abilities

Absorbent, picks up your energies, both positive and negative

Used for centering self; stimulates memory

Enhances intuition; emotional balancer; imagination

Emotional expressiveness; spontaneity; peace

Pearl:
Increases receptivity to spiritual perceptions

Balances left/right brain; balances emotions

Helps one focus attention; soothing; peaceful

Enhances personal integrity

Inspires honesty; wisdom

Peridot:
Aids in forgiveness; aligns subtle bodies

Emotionally calming

Increases clarity, patience, and positive outlook

Eases depression and releases tension

Increases intuitive awareness; prosperity

Diminishes spiritual fears and guilt

Helps open inner sight to the spiritual

Pyrite:
Shields from many forms of negative energy

Eases anxiety, depression, frustration

Grounding; helps keep one centered

Enhances emotional body; influences a more positive outlook

Promotes psychic development, learning, and perception

Encourages communication between the conscious and subconscious mind

Quartz Crystal: Amplifies energy; energizing; emotional balancer

Raises one's vibration; balances energy; stores and transmits energy

Dispels negativity; encourages positive thoughts

Shields from many forms of negative energy

Often used for meditating and enhancing intuition

Frequently used for spiritual healing; receiving guidance

Promotes harmony and understanding; amplifies thought-forms

Spiritual development; maximizes prayers and wishes

Quartz Clusters: Breaks up negative energies in an environment

Quartz, Rose: Increases creativity and self-expression

Enhances self-confidence

Used to communicate with nature spirits

Transmits and focuses energy; helps heal emotional pain

Encourages us to be peaceful, loving, and gentle

Helps us attract positive love into our lives; enhances self-love

Promotes positive outlook; teaches forgiveness and tolerance

Helps clear stored anger, resentment, guilt, fear, and jealousy

Reduces stress and tension; calms the nerves

Aligns mental, emotional, and astral bodies

Emanates unconditional love and nurturance

Heals the heart and reassures

Quartz, Rutilated: Enhances life force and insight; communication with Higher Self

Brings subconscious patterns to the conscious mind for examination

Stimulates the electrical properties in the body

Facilitates inspiration and happiness; eases depression

Transmutes negativity; opens crown for meditation

More intensity than clear quartz; clairvoyance; telepathy

Promotes determination, self-control, and strength of will

Quartz, Smoky: Promotes serenity and calmness; Higher Guidance

Often used in centering and grounding energy

Eases depression, fear, and panic; clears the aura

Helps in divination and creativity

Stabilizing; alleviates nightmares; aids grief

Improves intuition; facilitates meditation

Works well with root chakra to release negative blocks

Enhances positive attitudes

Rhodocrosite: Soothes and heals emotions; increases energy levels

Strengthens self-identity; aligns subtle bodies;

Cleanses subconscious mind, allowing higher realms of thought

Unites the conscious and subconscious

Helps ease extreme trauma, inner child issues; helps loneliness

Inspires forgiveness; helps develop compassion

Bridges upper and lower chakras; assists healing of heart center

Enhances memory and intellectual power

Assists with developing psychic growth

Facilitates self-forgiveness and self-love

Rhodonite: Eases physical/emotional trauma; improves memory

Develops greater sensitivity

Raises feeling of self-worth and stability; confidence

Alleviates anxiety and confusion; reduces stress; calms mind

Soothes nightmares

Strengthens mantra use, chanting, affirmation, and toning

Helps us see both sides of the issue; tolerance

Ruby:

Intensifies all emotions; energizes

Courage; integrity; stamina; vitality

Intuition is enhanced; spiritual devotion and spiritual wisdom

Eases disappointment, grief, and melancholia

Helps mental concentration; leadership ability

Fosters integrity, enthusiasm, generosity, and happiness

Sapphire:

Mental stabilizer and very grounding; insight; intuition; wisdom

Helps with organization and self-discipline

Dispels confusion; calms nerves

Counteracts mental depression

Excellent for meditation; amplifies intuitive abilities

Brings joy and peace of mind; creative expression; happiness

Selenite:

Soothes emotions; enhances will power

Activates spiritual insight; aids concentration and clarity

Expands sensitivity and field of awareness

May help physical and emotional letting go; meditation

Draws out negative thought patterns and replaces them with peace

Psychic development; positive thoughts; emotional flexibility

Sodalite:

Heals emotional and stress-related diseases

Stills the mind and promotes wisdom

Releases anger and fear; awakens third eye

Fosters learning proficiency and self-expression

General communication and writing aid

Eases subconscious guilt

Helps keep mind clear and rational

Sugilite: Third-eye activator; reduces stress

Enhances sensitivity and conscious awareness; excellent for meditation

Opens the connection between mind and body; cleanses the aura

Activates and balances brain hemispheres

Helps to deflect negative energies

Develops psychic awareness; peace of mind

Absorbs and dissolves anger; alleviates depression

Increases vibrational rate to absorb higher frequencies more easily

Helps one relinquish negative thoughts

Tiger Eye: Focuses thought and enhances intuition; confidence

Aids in clarity of perception; emotional balancer

Helps one see and understand different perspectives

Encourages psychic and intuitive knowledge

Protects against negative forces; centering; grounding

Clears mental confusion; assists decision-making

Helps separate thoughts from feelings

Enhances personal empowerment; courage

Integrates male and female energy within us

Calms emotions; aids meditation

Topaz: Revitalizes energy; grounding; mental clarity; personal power

Protects against insomnia and depression

Helps to balance emotions and eliminate mood swings

Develops psychic abilities; perceptivity; inspiration; peacefulness

Increases imagination; connects all the different energy centers

Draws negativity from chakras

Encourages confidence in trusting one's decisions

Tourmaline: Balances energies of the lower chakras with the higher chakras

Works as a protective shield; deflects negative energy

Aligns subtle bodies

Helps in grounding spiritual energies; concentration; inspiration

Dispels fear and negativity; bestows self-confidence

Calms the nerves; enhances sensitivity and understanding

Transmutes lower-frequency energy to a higher frequency of light

Allows us to be flexible and tolerant

Tourmaline, Pink: Disperses emotional pain and old destructive feelings

Promotes peace; inspires trust in love

Turquoise: Uplifting; increases sensitivity; fostering of empathy

Attracts wealth; aligns chakras

Enhances meditation; encourages positive thinking

Assists emotional balance; grounding

Excellent for healing of energy centers and the physical body

Helps us to see more clearly physically and spiritually

Increases creativity and imagination; brings peace of mind

Dissipates negativity; induces wisdom and understanding

Opens heart center; serenity

PLEASE NOTE: If you are drawn to a particular crystal (or stone), then that is the vibration that your spirit is requesting. Also, if you lose a crystal or have the urge to pass it on, please don't worry—it simply means that you no longer have the need for it. A new one will soon replace it.

Grounding Stones
Agate
Amber
Bloodstone
Boji stone
Carnelian
Chrysoprase
Fluorite
Garnet
Hematite
Jade
Jasper
Malachite
Obsidian
Onyx
Petrified wood
Pyrite
Smoky quartz
Sapphire
Tiger eye
Topaz
Tourmaline
Turquoise

Meditation Stones
Amethyst
Aquamarine
Azurite
Celestite
Chrysocolla
Chrysoprase
Fluorite
Herkimer diamond
Howlite
Jade
Kyanite

Lapis
Moonstone
Pearl
Clear quartz
Rutilated quartz
Smoky quartz
Selenite
Sugilite
Turquoise

Spiritual Development Stones
Amethyst
Citrine
Celestite
Kunzite
Kyanite
Clear quartz
Rhodochrosite
Selenite
Sugilite
Sodalite
Topaz

Peaceful Stones
Amethyst
Aquamarine
Chrysocolla
Lapis
Jade
Rose quartz
Malachite
Kyanite
Kunzite
Selenite
Turquoise

Protection Stones
Agate
Alexandrite
Citrine
Crystal cluster
Fluorite
Labradorite
Malachite
Sardonyx
Tiger eye
Turquoise

Healing Stones
Amber
Amethyst
Aventurine
Azurite
Citrine
Clear quartz
Rhodochrosite
Rutilated quartz
Turquoise
Water tourmaline

Favorite Prayers

The power of holy prayers of any world religion to which you are most attuned can assist you in elevating your vibrational frequencies. Prayer is the act of talking to Source.[40] For your spiritual progression, it would be beneficial to become aware of which spiritual words, music, and prayers resonate most with you. These prayers can assist in transforming your mental system as well as your entire four-body system. By saying such prayers or chanting mantras, you are using the word as a co-creator with Source, intoning the highest possible vibrational frequencies.[41]

This prayer comes straight out of the Bible and is probably the most widely known prayer in Christianity.

The Lord's Prayer

Our Father, Who art in heaven, Hallowed be thy name.
Thy Kingdom Come, Thy Will be done on Earth as it is in Heaven.
Give us this day our daily bread,
And forgive us our debts as we forgive our debtors.
And lead us not into temptation, but deliver us from evil.
For Thine is the Kingdom and the Power and the Glory, forever.[42]

The Great Invocation

The Great Invocation is a World Prayer, an invocation to Light and Love, and is used globally as a service to humanity. The Invocation does not belong to any person or group, but to all humanity. Tens of thousands of people of goodwill throughout the world recite it daily. It can be used regardless of background or creed and is translated into almost seventy languages and dialects.

There are two versions of this prayer. The original was released in 1945 by Alice Bailey and the Tibetan Djwhal Khul. The newer version that follows was adapted in 2000 by the Lucis Trust to accommodate the world's changing consciousness.[43]

The Great Invocation

From the point of Light within the Mind of God
Let light stream forth into human minds.
Let Light descend on Earth.
From the point of Love within the Heart of God
Let love stream forth into human hearts.
May the Coming One *return to Earth.*
From the center where the Will of God is known
Let purpose guide all little human wills,
The purpose which the Masters know and serve.
From the center which we call the human race
Let the Plan of Love and Light work out
And may it seal the door where evil dwells.
Let Light and Love and Power
restore the Plan on Earth.[44]

The next prayer was written by James Dillet Freeman for all soldiers during World War II. It is as powerful today as it was then.[45]

Unity Prayer of Protection

The light of God surrounds me;
The love of God enfolds me;
The power of God protects me;
The presence of God watches over me;
Wherever I am, God is!

The Soul Mantram

This powerful ancient mantra was brought forth to the Earth through the channelings of Alice Bailey and the Ascended Master Djwhal Khul, to activate the help of your soul. When spoken aloud, each of the statements of affirmation produces certain results in the subtle bodies that clear and energize them. It is also believed that saying this prayer, prior to any spiritual practice, will ignite your Higher Self and I AM Presence.

Soul Mantram

(Repeat three times aloud)

I AM the Soul,

I AM the Light Divine,

I AM Love,

I AM Will,

I AM Fixed Design.[46]

The Gayatri Mantra

The Gayatri Mantra has been revered for thousands of years and is one of the holiest mantras of the Hindu religion. It is an equivalent of The Lord's Prayer in Christianity. It is called "The Mantra of Spiritual Light." It is believed to heal the body, feed the Spirit, and illumine the mind.[47]

Most chant the Gayatri Mantra daily. However, the ideal times for chanting the mantra are three times a day—at dawn, midday, and dusk. These times are known as the three *sandhyas*. It is said that the maximum benefit of chanting the mantra is obtained by chanting it 108 times. However, one may chant it for 3, 9, or 18 times if time is a concern.[48]

The following is one of the many interpretations of this sacred prayer.

O Thou Who givest sustenance to the universe,

From Whom all things proceed,

To Whom all things return,

Unveil to us the face of the true Spiritual Sun

Hidden by a disc of golden Light

That we may know the Truth and do our whole duty

As we journey to Thy sacred feet.

Prayers for Strength

The next two prayers are ones that I have personally turned to over the years when undergoing challenges of many types. It was not unusual for me to repeat them many times a day for several months in a row.[49]

In My Weakest Moment

The place on which I am standing right now is Holy Ground.
I am standing in the midst of my own personal spiritual transformation, and it is unfolding perfectly.
In the midst of my most difficult lesson, I am gaining strength, growing in power, increasing in wisdom, and being fulfilled in every need.
In my weakest moment, I am faced with a divine opportunity for God to demonstrate just how awesome the power of God is in me.
I know this to be true.
I accept this to be true.
Right now, right where I am, the experience and expression of the truth I need to know is manifesting perfectly.
What a blessing! And So It Is!

Prayer of Surrender

Dear God:
Today I acknowledge, accept, and admit that my life is a God-job, and I surrender my life to you.
Today, I surrender fear, doubt, worry, anxiety, and control.
Today, I acknowledge, accept, and admit that I cannot fix anyone or anything.
Today, I acknowledge, accept, and admit that I cannot heal anyone or anything.
Today, I acknowledge, accept, and admit that I cannot help anyone.
Today, I acknowledge, accept, and admit that I cannot control anyone or anything.
Today, I acknowledge, accept, and admit that I cannot fix, change, heal, or help myself.
I am a God-job. My life is a God-job.
Today, dear God, please have your perfect way with me, for I know that the least you can be to me and for me is good.
For this I am so grateful!
And So It Is!

Light Invocation

This short daily prayer is not attached to any religion. It allows any individual to call forth and activate the Divine Light that is the basis of all faiths:

> *I invoke the Light of the Source within. I AM a clear and perfect channel. Light is my guide.*[50]

The Mantram of Unification

This mantram is a source of strength for all disciples active in spiritual work. It was originally published in 1955 in the book *Discipleship in the New Age, Vol. 2,* by the Tibetan Master Djwhal Khul, through his Channel, Alice A. Bailey.

> *The sons of men are one and I am one with them.*
>
> *I seek to love, not hate;*
> *I seek to serve and not exact due service;*
> *I seek to heal, not hurt.*
>
> *Let pain bring due reward of light and love.*
> *Let the soul control the outer form, and life and all events*
> *And bring to light the love that underlies the happenings of the time.*
>
> *Let vision come and insight.*
> *Let the future stand revealed.*
> *Let inner union demonstrate and outer cleavages be gone.*
> *Let love prevail. Let all men love.*

Here we have a marvelous summation of the Divine Plan for man. To whatever extent we, as individuals, understand it and live by it, we aid the whole of humanity. It brings meaning and purpose to our lives.[51]

Peace Prayer of St. Francis

This prayer and affirmation of Saint Francis is one of the most beautiful prayers. It can be repeated aloud or silently. This prayer is attributed traditionally to St. Francis of Assisi (1181–1226).[52]

Lord, make me an instrument of Your peace;
Where there is hatred, let me sow love;
Where there is injury, pardon;
Where there is doubt, faith;
Where there is despair, hope;
Where there is darkness, light;
And where there is sadness, joy.

Say it each day three times, and expect a miracle of transformation.

———

By means of invocation, prayer, and meditation, divine energies can be released and brought into activity. Men and women of goodwill of many faiths and nations can join in world service, bringing spiritual value and strength to a troubled world. May the prayers above inspire you to include any of them in your daily spiritual practice.[53]

Chapter 8

Spiritual Ecology

Just as your health and well-being depend on balanced nutritional and fitness habits, your spiritual practices must also be in balance to promote total spiritual harmony. Ecology is about interactions and adaptations to your life processes and environment, and "spiritual ecology" incorporates the choices you make to promote your spiritual growth. Consistency is the key. To begin, it is important that you assess and accept where you actually are in your spiritual development. Once you have acknowledged where you are stuck in your life, you can formulate a plan for your healing and recovery. Awareness creates choice. Simply through your intention and focus, you can develop a more meaningful and positive life. Remember that this is a *process,* as there are no magic wands or fast tracks that can turn a life around in a split second. Rather, this is a journey to wholeness. After the realization has been reached that you are stuck in some level of your life the next step is to develop a vision or blueprint of what you now desire your life plan to be.

Daily Practice

According to Ruth Haley Barton in her book *Sacred Rhythms,* establishing a regular routine of spiritual practices takes some time and planning. It takes a while to explore a variety of disciplines so you have some sense of their relevance to you and how you might be able to incorporate them in a meaningful manner in your daily life. The best method to implement daily spiritual sessions is to explore each discipline individually for a time in order to discover how well it resonates with what you wish to achieve. No two individuals will have exactly the same rhythm, because no two people are alike nor have the same spiritual inclinations.[1]

It doesn't matter how structured or unstructured your chosen routine of spiritual practice, you must remember to maintain flexibility. It doesn't matter how much you organize your day, life will still happen that doesn't fit into your plan. Some prefer to begin the day focused in spirituality, and others will choose to end the day in that manner. Whichever basic rhythm of spiritual practice you choose, you gain the most benefit by committing fully to it.

This commitment might require rearranging your present daily schedule and/or communicating with family or friends about your spiritual intentions and time and space requirements. Research has shown that it takes thirty days to establish a habit. Use whatever amount of time is available at first, but commit to a consistent time of day for your focus and intention. Gradually you will choose to increase the allocated amount of time as you strive for spiritual growth and wholeness.

Once your choices have been determined, you can begin to create a spiritual practice on a daily basis that will provide you with focus, support, sustenance, and creativity for other possibilities. This can be accomplished through daily prayer, meditations, spiritual CDs and books, music, yoga, singing, chanting, or breathing. Additionally, it is of utmost importance to start and/or close your day with gratitude for all the positive experiences that are in your life on all levels. In Chrissie Blaze's book *Workout for the Soul,* she outlines a fifteen-minute daily workout that could easily be woven into a person's everyday routine; it includes a Violet Flame visualization.[2]

Ideas for creating a daily practice: There are many different exercises included in this book. Choose one at a time and work with the exercise for a period of time rather than attempting to experience all of them at once. If you do not see or feel something changing, just know that it is happening through your intention. Sometimes it is only in retrospect that you realize changes have occurred.

The best way to start and maintain a spiritual practice is to incorporate it into your daily routine. To begin, schedule a set time once or twice a day for your practice. You may find that it is easier to stick with your practice if you do it first thing in the morning before you get engaged in other tasks and responsibilities. You will glean the most from your daily spiritual practice if you are fully awake and alert. Eventually you will choose to increase the allotted amount of time as you strive for spiritual wholeness. There is no single method that is best. The right choice is one that resonates with you and fits your lifestyle.

- Radiate Divine love into the world from your heart via your intention each day.
- Place yourself and family members daily in the tri-colored bubbles of protection.
- Take a two-minute breathing break several times a day.
- Exercise daily—do whatever makes you happy.
- Listen to guided imagery.
- Spend time in nature in silence daily.
- Read books on angels.
- Evoke the Violet Transmuting Flame into parks, schools, and hospitals.
- Play inspirational and spiritual music.
- Use meditation and prayer often.

Frequent contact with spirit guides will result in improvement in all phases of your life, quicker manifestations of your prayers, and your becoming a more open and loving being to others.

The good news about the journey of spiritual evolution is that you cannot go backward on your spiritual path though you can stay stuck or move upward. In order to attract good things into your life, you must become aware of the frequency at which you are vibrating. This can be discovered by observing your emotions, your environment, and your relationships.

Below are various options for creating a realistic daily spiritual practice to interface with your personal responsibilities.

Beginning

1. Deep Breathing

With its focus on full, cleansing breaths, deep breathing is a simple yet powerful inner-focus method. All you need is a few minutes and a place to stretch out. The key is to breathe deeply from the abdomen, getting as much fresh air as possible into your lungs. Put one hand on your chest and the other hand on your abdomen. Breathe in through your nose, and as you do, the hand on your abdomen should rise. Then exhale through your mouth, pushing out as much air as you can while contracting your abdominal muscles. Continue this process for three to five minutes. You might choose to take a two-minute breathing break several times a day.

2. Tapping Thymus

Tapping the area over your thymus will stimulate all of your energies, boost your immune system, and increase your strength and vitality. This technique can help you if you are feeling overwhelmed by negative energies, starting to get a cold, fighting an infection, or your immune system is compromised in some manner. Begin by locating your thymus gland approximately two inches below the notch of your throat. Gently tap the thymus for approximately one to two minutes. It is also is very advantageous to tap your thymus point when you are under stress.

3. Focus on Your Heart Center

Place your dominant hand over your heart and imagine that you can breathe in and out from that area for a few seconds. As you do, become quiet in your mind and concentrate on the word "LOVE." Think in terms of radiating love out into your environment and then to family members or to anyone you wish to send loving or healing thoughts. Consciously sit and radiate love and blessings into your home and then to the Earth. You might take two or three minutes, morning and evening, to radiate love to others while you focus your attention upon your Heart Center.

4. Meditate

Choosing one of the varieties of techniques listed in Chapter 11, "The Empowerment of Meditation," allow yourself five to fifteen minutes of inner stillness. Many of the skills in meditation can apply to daily activities. For example, you can meditate when you are on a plane, train, or bus, or while waiting in line.

5. Send Healing to the Earth

For a few moments, visualize our beautiful planet and imagine it being totally engulfed in Violet Fire and cleansed and purified. Also, you can use some of the meditations at the end of this book for cleansing the Earth daily.

6. Gratitude

Don't get out of bed until you say a dozen things for which you are thankful and appreciative of in life. Be grateful for everyone who has been there for you.

7. Recite a mantra, decree affirmation, or prayer three times aloud.

Some examples would be:

I AM that I AM
Om Mani Padme Hum (Mantra of Compassion)
Shalom (Peace)
The Lord's Prayer
Hail Mary
Om Shanti (Mantra of Peace)
The Soul Mantram
The Great Invocation
Word Mantras such as: Peace, Joy, Love, Harmony, Tolerance, Compassion, Balance, Oneness

8. Bed Cleansing

Since considerable emotional release takes place during your sleep state, it would be beneficial to call forth the Violet Transmuting Flame every day to transmute old or lingering energies when you awaken each morning. Your aura is like a magnet and picks up vibrational energies that are floating around everywhere you go. It is therefore important to cleanse your aura on a daily basis as well. One way to do this is to visualize this Violet Fire pouring into your physical body and filling every cell. Then request that this Violet Fire move through your emotional, mental, and etheric bodies separately.

9. Protection

State aloud:

I command that a bubble be placed around me and that Blue Light stream through and immerse this entire bubble, forming a grid on the interior of the bubble. I command that Gold Light stream through the bubble, continuing to form the grid, and I command that Pink Light stream through and immerse this entire space now.

I command that Violet Light fill this entire bubble, transmuting all misqualified energy, and that all remnants be sent to the Light to be requalified now.

I command that all energy that is no longer for the highest good be released and sent to the Light now.

I command that only those energies that are for the highest good be allowed to exist within this bubble from this point forward.

I command that love, joy, peace, clarity, harmony, wisdom, trust, creativity, abundance, perfect health, humility, faith, as well as every other divine quality that is for my highest good, radiate permanently from this grid and throughout this entire bubble.

I command that only the Beings of Light may change these commands to bring about an even greater good.

So be it. So be it. So be it.

10. Chant OM

This can be done aloud or as a silent chant within the heart and soul.

Intermediate

1. Light Meditation to Build the Inner Shrine
2. Recite the Great Invocation
3. Say the Soul Mantram
4. Meditate for twenty minutes
5. Perform one or two yoga asanas or body stretches
6. Radiate LOVE into the world from your heart each day
7. The I AM Technique
8. Balance your chakras
9. Align your will with the will of Source, through intention
10. Radiate Violet Fire within, around, and through the Earth and especially after horrific events

Increasing Vibrations

Your personal vibration is the overall frequency that radiates from you all the time. This vibration is a combination of all aspects of your body, your emotions, and your thoughts. It naturally fluctuates according to your moods.[3] It is your unique vibratory signature in the Universe.

Thought vibrations are continually present. We attract the current that harmonizes with us. The more pure, sincere, and positive our thoughts, the higher will be the rate of vibration. Your personal vibration is created by your choices, thoughts, and actions. The more you allow your Spirit to shine through, the higher the personal vibration that you generate.[4] When you have a higher vibration, there is more spiritual energy in your body. Increasing your vibrations will raise the quality of your soul's energy. In order to accelerate the vibratory action of your inner bodies, it is important that you consciously draw Light into them. The Light will act similar to an electric charger as it flows into each electron, causing it to spin more rapidly in its orbit as it moves around the center of the atom. It is sustained by conscious effort through decree work, visualizations, and prayers, and also by constant vigilance over the type of feelings you store in your emotional body and the type of thoughts you dwell upon.

In order to refine and purify your emotional body, it is necessary to use the Violet Fire through it constantly.[5]

You are surrounded by a plethora of energy vibrations in your environment, from electromagnetic frequencies, to vibrations of sound and temperature, to basic waves of matter. Some vibrations are perceived via your senses, but the majority are not. Your personal vibration is affected by the vibrations of other people and the vibrations of the world, and who you want to be. However, how you want to feel is your choice.[6] Since life is short, learning to enjoy each and every present moment is not that difficult.[7] It is a mindset that you consciously choose each and every moment of every day.

Eating the Rainbow

According to Gabriel Cousens, MD, holistic health physician, "the vibrations of food are first absorbed visually." Consequently, Dr. Cousens recommends that we embrace the Rainbow Diet. In the Rainbow Diet system, all foods have a vibrational connection to the seven main chakras and their colors, and these correspond to the spectrum of the rainbow. Also, differently colored foods are specific for energizing, balancing, and healing their specific color-related chakras. At the same time, each color-related food energizes, cleanses, builds, heals, and rebalances the glands, organs, and nerve centers associated with its color-related chakra. The purpose of the Rainbow Diet is to help balance, on a regular daily cycle, each chakra, its associated organs, glands, and nerve plexus, and the chakra system as a whole. This concept is based on mostly vegetarian food: vegetables, fruits, nuts, seeds, grains, along with eggs and dairy products. Research has shown that food is energy. Scientists have found that each food has a specific energy frequency and resonance field.[8]

A capsule summary of the Rainbow Diet is: eat a full spectrum of foods for the full spectrum of the chakras throughout the spectrum of the day. The morning addresses the first three chakras: red, orange, and yellow. Midday is the third through fifth chakras: yellow-gold, green, and blue in color. Evening focuses on the fifth through seventh chakras:

blue, indigo, and violet-purple. In this diet, white foods (which represent the full rainbow spectrum) can be eaten at any meal.[9] You could say that the Rainbow Diet functions as a support system to aid a harmonious spiritual unfolding. If you want more information about the basics of this diet and the timing of meals, I suggest that you obtain a copy of Dr. Cousens's book, *Spiritual Nutrition and the Rainbow Diet*.

Besides striving to eat fruits and vegetables in all shades of the rainbow, consider the following in your nutritional choices: Ideally, purchase fresh produce that is seasonal, locally grown, and organic, when possible. The further removed that the food is from its source, the fewer nutrients it will have for your body. Choose whole, unrefined, and unprocessed foods and eat them raw when appropriate. Then pay attention to your level of satiety and stop eating when you are 80% satisfied, but not full.

The Great Invocation Full-Moon Program

This ancient prayer is especially powerful if it is chanted within a five-day period of a full moon. By chanting it aloud thirteen continuous times, you complete one cycle. To gain the full momentum of the influence of the full-moon time frame, thirteen cycles (13x13) per day must be said over a five-day period. This thirteen-per-day cycle must be chanted the two days before the full moon, then the day of the actual full moon, and then for two days after the full moon occurs. Years ago, I recorded my thirteen-per-day chants on a cassette tape, which I mentally said in accompaniment as it played on my tape recorder. Now people can record on their MP3 devices or their cell phones, if they wish. Working with the Great Invocation in the way described below will give you a high-frequency boost and increase your vibrational field.[10]

Start first thing in the morning of day one. Say the Great Invocation aloud thirteen times, one after another as a gentle continuous chant, which makes one cycle. You then repeat this cycle another twelve times during that day, making a total of thirteen cycles in all for one day. Then repeat this full day's program of thirteen cycles on each day over the next four days, making a five-day program for that full moon. This five-day program is repeated over the next twelve consecutive full moons, making a total program spanning thirteen full moons for the year.

Initially you may think this program requires too much discipline and dedication. So let me explain the reasons fulfilling the thirteen-moon cycle is important. Then your Higher Self may nudge you into making the necessary commitments. The discipline needed to complete this program over a continuous thirteen-moon cycle is worth the effort as you enhance your energy pattern, amplify your circuitry, and bring together any vibrational fragmentation in your body. This will increase your capacity to handle and hold energy, raise your vibration, and move you into a whole new tempo.[11]

The text of the Great Invocation appears in Chapter 7, under the section entitled "Favorite Prayers."

Chapter 9

Angelic Soul Recovery

Traditionally the practice of soul retrieval or recovery is implemented by trained shamans. They enter into an altered state of consciousness to access other dimensions to recover soul parts. Not having any type of shamanism training, I decided to ask my Higher Self about the possibility of retrieving my own soul fragments by partnering with angels. Angelic Soul Recovery is the technique that I then channeled through my automatic writing in order to reintegrate various parts of my soul that might have become disconnected, trapped, or lost through trauma.

I originally requested this process from the Universe when I moved to Sedona, Arizona, in 1992. I was newly married but felt like something was missing. Since I was a Certified Clinical Hypnotherapist at the time, I performed several past-life regressions on myself. As a result, I recalled several lifetimes with tragic situations whereby I could have experienced soul fragmentation or loss. Since I was not trained as a shaman but felt comfortable working in conjunction with the Angelic realm, this process in this chapter was revealed to me. After this book you are holding was written, I was guided to incorporate the information in this chapter to empower you to recover any soul pieces or splinters that would assist you as you journey to your Ascension.

Soul fragmentation happens when an individual's essence, also known as the soul, experiences a serious trauma, mental or physical abuse, tremendous pain, or drama during a lifetime, which causes a piece of the soul to tear or splinter. The basic premise is that whenever we experience trauma, a part of our vital essence separates from us in order to survive by escaping the full impact of the pain. Soul loss can be caused by whatever a person experiences as traumatic—even if another person would not experience it that way. Shamanic belief is that part of our essential life energy can split off and become lost in "nonordinary reality." Some of the symptoms of this phenomenon are:

1. A gap in memory, such as no recall of one's life from ages seven to nine (for example), or twelve to fourteen.

2. A shock or emotional jolt. The reaction might be normal for the situation, but for some reasons the part of Self that left fails to return.

3. Chronic depression can occur. After the fragment leaves, the person is kept from being able to create a path of joy. Instead he or she feels depressed and unfulfilled.

4. Divorce or death creates periods of grief. If a person didn't recover from the emotional trauma of separation, a piece of the soul might be lost.

5. Physical illness can also be a symptom of soul loss. Often when we give our power away, we become ill.

6. Numbness, apathy, and emptiness are also symptoms.[1]

In some way, most of us experience some degree of soul loss. Some people have been more deeply traumatized by life. For some people, this feeling of incompleteness and alienation causes great suffering.

In our modern society and medical establishment, the soul fragmentation known to the ancient shamanic warriors is not acknowledged or understood. Instead, the symptoms are too often controlled by drugs in this physical world. Many who have soul fragmentation are placed upon medication, which quiets the emotions but does not help the cause of the troubles. It is of the utmost importance that the understanding of the soul not be lost in our present time. For it is the power within us and the nature of who we are. Those who experience continual loss of jobs, money, and homes are often suffering from soul loss. Those who experience continual suicide tendencies have lost pieces of themselves. There are many ways a soul can become fragmented, but the most convincing sign is the loss of power within a person's life.

You may not know for sure if your soul has lost fragments, but if you feel there might be a slight chance, you will be wise to explore the possibility of the Angelic Soul Recovery process. It has been understood from past experiences that it can take up to six weeks for the returned soul parts to be integrated fully into the whole.

A Checklist of Soul-Loss Symptoms

The following questions are excerpted from Sandra Ingerman's book *Soul Retrieval*. They are helpful in determining whether soul loss has occurred. To see whether soul loss is an issue for you and, if so, how it manifests in your life, ask yourself the following questions:

1. Do you ever have a difficult time staying "present" in your body? Do you sometimes feel as if you are outside your body observing it as you would a movie?

2. Do you ever feel numb, apathetic, or deadened?

3. Do you suffer from chronic depression?

4. Do you have problems with your immune system and have trouble resisting illness?

5. Were you chronically ill as a child?

6. Do you have gaps in memory of your life after age five? Do you have a sense that you may have blacked out significant traumas in your life?

7. Do you struggle with addictions to (for example) alcohol, food, sex, or gambling?

8. Do you find yourself looking for external things to fill up emptiness?

9. Have you had difficulty moving on with your life after a divorce or a death?

10. Do you suffer from multiple personality disorder?

If you answer "yes" to any of these questions, you may be dealing with soul loss. Important parts of your essential core self may not be available to you. If so, the vital energy and gifts of these parts are temporarily inaccessible.[2]

Descriptions of Soul Fragmentation

People describe the condition of soul fragmentation in the following ways, as excerpted from *Healing Lost Souls* by William Baldwin:

- "Spacey"
- "All broken up"
- "Shattered"
- "Falling apart"
- "My senses feel dead"
- "Out to lunch"
- "Nobody home"
- "Not playing with a full deck"
- "Brokenhearted"
- "He stole my heart"
- "Airheaded"
- "Feel like I'm being torn apart"
- "Need to pull myself together"
- "Not firing on all cylinders"
- "One foot in the grave"
- "Need to get my head together"
- "Empty-headed"
- "Don't feel whole"
- "Feel out of kilter, out of balance"
- "Part of me says 'yes,' part of me says 'no'"
- "Need to gather my thoughts"

These common idioms may seem like meaningless slang, yet they are often clear metaphorical descriptions of problems by people who have suffered soul fragmentation.[3]

Preparation for Soul-Recovery Process

1. First you must assess what soul percentage you are now missing. When you ask yourself this percentage question, it is vital that you accept the very first number that pops into your awareness, no matter how outrageous it may seem: "What percentage of my soul is missing?" Immediately write that percentage in the upper right corner of the Soul Recovery Assessment form that follows.

2. Next, discern when and where any soul loss might have occurred. Briefly, meditate on what geographical locations you are fond of, as well as what cultures and eras of time you resonate with. Then list each separately on the Soul Recovery Assessment sheets (below). If you have skills dowsing, then you can obtain more specific answers.

3. Then list the events, geographical areas, or historical time periods under Part One, Two, Three, etc., where you might have had soul parts leave you. For each of those situations, discern who in your non-physical or spiritual life you would want to journey to other dimensions to retrieve those soul fragments. These Beings will be listed for each missing soul part on the "Volunteer" line on the Soul Recovery Assessment form.

4. Review the Checklist of Soul-Loss Symptoms (above) to determine what symptoms you may be experiencing.

5. Obtain a medium-sized clear quartz crystal. The crystal is the receptacle where the soul fragments are placed by the Beings of Light to hold all the splinters and fragments together when they are returned. The crystal serves as a "Soul Catcher," like a comfortable holding space for the soul parts.

This crystal is especially helpful if the soul has shattered—it acts as a vacuum cleaner to sweep up the splintered parts.

Make copies of the following pages to use during any soul recoveries, though one or two sessions is enough for most people.

Soul-Recovery Assessment

When a soul part is recovered, it always brings a gift when it returns. This is usually in the form of a characteristic or an ability. It is not necessary to know what that will be until the soul part is integrated into an individual. The following worksheet will help you document what you experience during your soul-recovery session.

Date: _____ Percentage Missing: _____

Part One: _____
    Volunteer: _____
    Ability to: _____

Part Two: _____
    Volunteer: _____
    Ability to: _____

Part Three: _____
    Volunteer: _____
    Ability to: _____

Part Four: _____
    Volunteer: _____
    Ability to: _____

Part Five: _____
    Volunteer: _____
    Ability to: _____

Part Six: _____
    Volunteer: _____
    Ability to: _____

Part Seven: _____

    Volunteer: _____

    Ability to: _____

Part Eight: _____

    Volunteer: _____

    Ability to: _____

Part Nine: _____

    Volunteer: _____

    Ability to: _____

Part Ten: _____

    Volunteer: _____

    Ability to: _____

Part Eleven: _____

    Volunteer: _____

    Ability to: _____

Part Twelve: _____

    Volunteer: _____

    Ability to: _____

Part Thirteen: _____

    Volunteer: _____

    Ability to: _____

Recovering Your Own Soul Fragments

First you will spend some time completing the Soul Recovery Assessment (above).

    1. *Light a candle. Place the clear quartz crystal for the session next to it.*

    2. *Say aloud this Healing Prayer:*

Dear Mother—Father—God,

I ask to be cleared and cleansed with the White Christ Light, the Green Healing Light, and the Violet Transmuting Light.

For my highest good and within God's will I ask that all disharmonious vibrations be removed from me, sealed within their own Light, and returned to the Source for purification, never again to re-establish within me or anyone else.

I ask that this room be surrounded by 100% pure Light, and that I be surrounded by Light. I ask for the protection of the triple shield of White Light of the Universal Protection. At this time I accept those forces of healing that work through and with me, which are only of 100% pure·Light.[4]

Then allow yourself to relax. Close your eyes and take four deep breaths, counting from one to four. Exhale slowly from each breath by counting backward from eight to one. Take a moment to scan your body, paying attention to any place where you are experiencing pain or tension.

Breathe deeply into any areas that are blocked, and take your time doing this so you can allow your body to relax fully. Imagine that you are in one of your favorite places out in nature, and use all your senses to notice what you are seeing and experiencing. Notice how you are feeling in this beautiful setting. Now find a comfortable place to lie down. When you do, take another very deep breath.

1. *Invoke the Spiritual Clearing Team by stating the following aloud:*

Through my divinity of Light I now call forth:

My Guides, Teachers, and Angels of 100% Light
My I AM Presence
Source
Beloved Legions of Light
Master St. Germain
Archangel Michael and all his legions to the front of me
Archangel Raphael and all his legions to the right of me
Archangel Uriel and all his legions behind me
Archangel Gabriel and all his legions to the left of me
The Overlighting Deva of Healing

I ask for total healing of mind, body, and spirit of this returning soul part and ask for any remaining negativity that this soul part may have from its travels to be removed and transmuted before it is returned and integrated.

> 2. Preface: State aloud the following for each separate soul part recovered.

Past, present, future; throughout all realms, all creations, all universes (real or imagined) and known or unknown, I request the return of all my soul parts from non-ordinary reality and from other people who have stolen* them.

> 3. Ask the requested/assigned "volunteer" (the designated Being of Light) that you previously listed on the Soul Recovery Assessment to go and retrieve each soul part separately.
>
> 4. Once the part is retrieved, ask the "volunteer" to place the soul fragment into the crystal.
>
> 5. Then cleanse each different soul part separately from trauma by stating aloud:

I now call upon the Law of Grace to erase the cause, the core, the effect, the record, and the memory of any and all negativity permanently and completely in this soul part; past, present, future, and throughout all time, all realms, all creations, all universes, and all dimensions, real or imagined, known or unknown. I now:

- Release all judgments of self
- Release all judgments of others, and
- Claim grace

I ask for total healing of this returning soul part and ask for any remaining negativity that this soul part may have from its travels to be removed and transmuted before it is returned and integrated.

I now call upon the Ascended Master St. Germain to direct the Violet Transmuting Flame toward any remaining negativity, transmuting it into pure Light and Unconditional Love. I evoke the full gathered momentum of the Violet Transmuting Flame.

*Ask the forces of Archangel Michael for assistance with stolen parts.

When you have discerned (via visualization, intuition, or pendulum) that the soul fragment(s) have been completely cleansed by the Violet Fire, move on to the following step.

6. *Hold the crystal in front of your heart and request Source, or a Spiritual Being, to blow the returned soul part into your heart chakra, through the crystal. Then hold the crystal over the top of your head and request Source, or a Spiritual Being, to blow the returned soul part into your crown chakra, through the crystal. Tune into any sensations or visualizations as the soul fragment(s) enter your body. Place your hands on your solar plexus and absorb the returned essence into every cell of your body. Then ask Archangel Michael and your Higher Self to gather up the cleansed soul parts and integrate them easily and gently within your Being.*

7. *Seal your aura with the crystal by passing it around your body four times.*

8. *Pause a moment and with gratitude say: "Welcome home!"*

9. *Now return to the Preface at Step 4 and repeat the same process above for each separate soul fragment that is returned.*

10. *When all soul fragments have been returned, state the Cosmic Law of Forgiveness:*

I invoke the Cosmic Law of Forgiveness for myself.
I forgive myself for anything I have done to anyone and
I forgive anyone for anything they have done to me.
So be it, So be it, So be it!

11. *Thank the Spiritual Clearing Team, and with gratitude release all Beings of Light.*

12. *State the following aloud:*

I thank all the following Beings of 100% Light who assisted me with this Soul Recovery today.
My Guides, Teachers, and Angels of 100% Light
My I AM Presence
Source
Beloved Legions of Light

Master St. Germain
Archangel Michael and all his legions to the front of me
Archangel Raphael and all his legions to the right of me
Archangel Uriel and all his legions behind me
Archangel Gabriel and all his legions to the left of me
The Overlighting Deva of Healing

13. *Drink some water. Then do one of the Grounding Exercises below or, weather permitting, walk outside barefooted for a few minutes to connect to the Earth.*

Grounding Exercises

Heaven and Earth

- Get as comfortable as possible while sitting in a chair with your feet firmly on the floor.
- Imagine that you are a mighty tree, e.g., a grandfather oak or towering redwood.
- Visualize your roots dividing into two major sections.
- Send these roots down through your feet to the ground and anchor them in the bedrock at the Earth's core.
- As you inhale, imagine that you are drawing up vibrant and nurturing Earth energy. Give it a color, if you wish.
- Visualize this warm and secure Earth energy moving up through your feet into your legs and torso.
- Imagine that it is filling up your entire physical body and each chakra all the way to the top of your head.
- As you exhale, allow this energy to mix with the energy of the cosmos.
- Now imagine a radiating white light above the top of your head.
- Allow it to cascade into your body, as though your body were a glass vessel.
- Visualize this white light moving down from your feet into the core of the Earth.
- Repeat this complete cycle three or four times.

Cable Grounding

- Get as comfortable as you are able to while seated in a chair. Make sure your feet are flat on the floor.
- Imagine that you have a cable attached to each hip and another one attached to your tailbone.
- Visualize them dropping down through the floor into the very core of the Earth.
- Allow these cables to now be anchored firmly, with gigantic hooks, into the bedrock of the Earth.
- Imagine the feeling of a dense forest moving up through these cables into your feet and lower torso.
- Carry this "anchoring thought" with you through the day.

Alignment Exercise

- Start from a seated position with your feet flat on the ground and take three deep breaths.
- Focus your attention on your first chakra at the base of your spine. Notice that this is the center of gravity of your physical body.
- Now in your imagination, place all your chakras from the top of your head to the base of your spine into a vertically aligned column.
- Notice that once all the chakras are in this position, they turn into a huge cord of light.
- Allow this cord to move down through your body, feet, and the ground into the center of the Earth with the flow of gravity.
- Once the contact with the Earth has been achieved, slowly open your eyes.

Possibilities for Soul Fragmentation

Following are some abilities, traits, and characteristics that may have been fragmented in this lifetime or previous ones. These are not the only possibilities, but they are the most common ones I have discovered over the years of performing Soul Recovery for clients. Please use your intuition, or any dowsing technique, to more specifically discern your own needs.

self-esteem	patience	joy	feeling safe
trust	faith	grace	self-nurturing
protection	wisdom	compassion	self-expression
adventuresome	self-love	independence	tranquility
spirituality	spontaneity	loyalty	commitment
guidance	confidence	intuition	self-empowerment
integrity	humility	attention	discipline
self-identification	sensitivity	inner peace	creativity
security	self-forgiveness	being good enough	acceptance
decisiveness	empathy	discernment	responsibility for self
gratitude	to believe in oneself	tolerance	peacefulness
positivity	self-worth	to receive love	freedom
to give love	more energy	to remember	personal power
loving-kindness	determination	ability to know self	strength
courage	hope	to focus	boundaries
happiness	liberation	intelligence	simplicity
heartfulness	generosity	playfulness	humor
motivation	worthiness	belonging	devotion
non-attachment	abundance	motivation	forgiveness
intimacy	decision making	gratefulness	awareness
inspiration	appreciation	wonderment	stability
balance	clarity	desire	intention
pleasure	peace of mind	perseverance	endurance
to be carefree	vitality	success	enthusiasm
adaptability	flexibility	wholeness	truth
relaxation	responsibility	surrender	receptivity
to listen	openness	self-assurance	resourceful
productivity	charity	determination	composure
expansiveness	to honor self	harmony	reliability
fulfillment	innocence	to heal	musical abilities
to study	to teach	to receive	to know

Stolen Soul Parts

Sometimes a soul, or part of it, has been stolen by another person. This is often done out of ignorance rather than intent to harm. The main reason another soul is stolen is power.

A person who has a victim or martyr mentality (can include abused women, men, or children; compulsive givers; or those who are codependent) is constantly giving away her/his energy, time, focus, and self to those who are more than willing to take them. Similarly, individuals who feel they are unlovable, suffer from low self-esteem, or have shame issues and/or bad boundaries often give pieces of themselves away. Frequently, the "taker" is the spouse, a child, relative, friend, or sometimes a co-worker.[5]

Effects of Soul Recovery

Integration of the returned soul parts takes some time. It would be best to wait a month before deciding whether to perform another Soul Recovery for yourself. Some people relive memories according to their internal timing. Some memories surface when it is the right time and place. Some memories reveal themselves in dreams.

The effects of Soul Recovery vary widely, and there is no absolute way to predict what will happen for a particular individual. Soon after a Soul Recovery, people comment that they feel warm throughout their body and feel "filled up" or lighter. They are more in their bodies. People who feel depleted before the session often feel more energy, power, and strength immediately. They may also feel giddy or burst into tears. However, they usually feel more peaceful when they leave after the session.

When you bring a soul part back, it is time for the ego and the body to evolve again into harmony with all life. A soul part that returns might have certain knowledge a person needs such as trust, love, creativity, play, or self-confidence. Most people don't require many Soul Recovery sessions. After one or two, most people have back what they need to experience wholeness in their lives.

It is possible that we have all suffered some soul loss during the course of our lives, but that doesn't mean we all need Soul Recovery. Life after this process is about learning to live in the present fully.[6]

Chapter 10

Divine Guidance

A number of methods are employed to develop greater attunement to your Higher Self and Source. Several are discussed below. Inner guidance appears in many forms: telepathy, inner hearing, visualizations, and intuitive knowing. By spending time each day in silence, you will develop skills to receive the messages that will be communicated to you. True and positive inner guidance is always revealed by the results in your life when you follow it.[1]

Higher Self

Your Higher Self is a reflection of your soul, and you have known it in every lifetime you have experienced. It is the energy of one's True Self. Your Higher Self resides above your head, far enough away from the physical body to hear Divine wisdom clearly. You can perceive this spiritual part of yourself in many different ways. Each individual develops a connection in a manner that is unique to him or her. Some sense their Higher Self as energy, a feeling, or a color. Others experience this aspect as a wise sage or teacher or a nurturing and caring Being. Whatever the image, the reunion will be filled with joy and happiness. Your Higher Self is entrusted with the secret ideal blueprint of your unique individual design and will assist you in achieving it. This is the most important partner you can have in moving forward spiritually. It is the part of you that knows all the answers for your spiritual path. This non-physical part of you is not at all separate from you, even though you may feel as though you are detached from it. It is the integral aspect of yourself that remains aware of and interacts positively with the whole of your Being. It is always available to be called upon for guidance. It is your personal source of wisdom. Learning to access this inner guidance is dependent upon the level of spiritual growth you have attained, as it is your connection to Source. It is a spark of the Divine Mind.

Access to your Higher Self is contingent on the amount of intention and dedication you allocate on a daily basis to create alignment with it. It can be reached through the discipline of meditation or the focus of prayer. These practices coupled with a sincere desire to align with your Higher Self will allow you access to the reservoir of greater knowledge, awareness, and intuition. Eventually this aspect of you will be integrated into all that you interface with and accomplish. Ultimately this integration of your Higher Self is a process of developing harmony that will enrich your life on a daily basis.

In order to receive higher and more direct guidance from Divine wisdom, it is imperative that your vibrations be increased. Since your Higher Self vibrates at a higher rate than your current third-dimensional body, it is necessary to raise your vibratory frequency to achieve a more direct link to higher consciousness via not only your Higher Self, but also Angels of 100% pure Light, Archangels, and Ascended Masters. By shifting from a thought that is negative to one that is positive, you can raise your energy vibration and strengthen yourself and the immediate energy field. Through prayer, meditation, daily reading of uplifting and spiritual books, and chanting, your vibrations can be elevated and your awareness heightened. For these practices to be truly effective, they should be undertaken at the same time each and every day. This will allow you to consciously realign with the rhythm of the Universe. Often people will develop the ability to perceive information from different senses than they previously relied on. These might include clairvoyance (clear sight), clairaudience (clear sound), clairsentience (clear feeling), or claircognizance (clear knowing).

Automatic Writing

As I continued on my spiritual path, I became more fascinated with developing my psychic gifts. However, over the years no spiritual talents appeared. Even though I attended a plethora of workshops, seminars, and lectures, I eventually felt like I needed more connection with my own guidance. I no longer wanted to rely on other people's messages for me.

By the late 1980s, I had become a successful hypnotherapist in private practice. As such, I often practiced self-hypnosis to resolve some of my past issues and frequently recalled my past-life experiences. One day while studying for my Doctorate in hypnotherapy, I came upon a technique called automatic writing. It sounded intriguing to me so I decided to explore it further. Since I was not clairvoyant or clairaudient, and could not see or hear my spirit guides and angels, I needed to develop another method to receive guidance for my own spiritual expansion. Ultimately, automatic writing proved to be the answer to my personal quest. It enabled me to channel my Higher Self and thereby develop the psychic gift of claircognizance, which is a deep and automatic knowing of the truth. This communication skill is a practice that I still use to this day—for creativity, problem-solving, and guidance in spiritual development. Next to meditation, this technique of automatic writing has been the second most instrumental process in my spiritual progression. The definition of this process of divination is writing that is performed without the use of the conscious mind of the writer—that is, writing performed by the unconscious muscular energies of the hand and arm. The writer is unaware of what will be written, as in a trance-like state. This method of channeling is also referred to as direct writing, non-conscious writing, and inspirational writing. It can be performed via a keyboard or pen and paper. The latter is what I prefer, as I am neither a fast nor efficient typist.

If you are interested in pursuing automatic writing, you will need to decide if you want to learn the technique using a computer or a pen and paper. If you choose the keyboard route, it is easier to start first with pen and paper and switch over to the computer after you have established a connection.

Find a location where you will be without distractions. It is important that you take the time to practice while relaxed and without disturbances. To develop this skill, it is necessary that you start with a clear mind. If you have any doubts or apprehension at this point, then you need not continue further. Doubt creates many obstacles to your success.

It is best if you sit for no longer than a half hour daily. Limiting the time period will prevent you from losing track of time. Setting a timer can be very helpful so you can devote your attention to the task of automatic writing and not worry about other projects or keep an eye on the clock. If possible, always do the session around the same time of day. A regular time ensures more help from any angelic realms or spirit guides who are assisting you in writing. They will come to assist you at certain stated times more easily than if your attempts are carried out on an irregular basis.

It is wise to limit your sessions for the first week. Start slowly and become comfortable with the experience. To begin an automatic writing session, take a few moments and enter into a calm and relaxed state of mind. This can be accomplished by chanting, focused breathing, listening to music, saying a prayer, self-hypnosis, autogenics, or alternate nostril breathing, as explained in Chapter 11. This will serve to raise your vibrations for an easier connection. To ensure that you are communicating only with highly spiritual sources, it is important that you place yourself in a force field of protection. I suggest you use the Protective Pillar of Light, as described in Chapter 5, "Spiritual Protection." Now you are ready to summon your connection. The key here is to request to be connected only with angels, guides, and teachers that are of 100% pure Light, or your Higher Self. These will be highly evolved and loving energies.

When you notice or feel that connection, then you may state your question or intentions aloud. Practice and patience are required. It is helpful if you begin with basic questions about yourself, or those that can be answered with a simple "yes" or "no." I like to state the following before I start my session (and after I create a protective force field that encompasses me): *"I ask that my Higher Self take full command of me now."* Then I follow with this question: *"What wisdom do you have for me today?"* I write in a spiral notebook and keep my eyes closed during the entire session to help keep my receptivity more tuned. The downside to this choice is that I frequently end up with sentences that are written over other sentences, and they are often difficult to decipher later. Lastly, I choose to sit in a dimly lit room and I always use a gel pen, as it seems to flow easier for me when I am writing rapidly.

At this point, the process begins. Relax your hands and rest your hand and pen gently against the paper in a writing position. The best way is to hold the arm clear of a table, so that neither the wrist, nor the elbow, nor any part of the arm touches it. In this manner a certain amount of fatigue is soon induced in the arm. When this occurs, automatic writing tends to begin. Trust the first impressions that come to mind regardless of how insignificant they might seem. Try not to write anything consciously. Just let the thoughts flow without your mental interference. In a short time, you will see or know that slight movements or scrawling marks are appearing on the paper. With diligence and practice the marks become more consistent until they form letters, then words, and finally entire sentences are written out. Once your hand begins to write, do not stop the flow to read what is being written.

Don't get discouraged if this process takes several sessions to occur. There is a time adjustment in order to receive the higher vibrational levels of this type of communication. The more you use automatic writing, the easier and faster it becomes. At first the information received might seem like random thoughts or even nonsense. Many of the messages, especially in the beginning, will doubtlessly prove incoherent and disconnected, like dreams. Do not judge or interpret what you have written until you complete the session, as that will switch your thinking from the right-brain intuitive activity to the left-brain functions of logic and reason. No matter what is received while writing, do not be concerned with the aesthetics of presentation. The content is the key. Also, notice how you are feeling during this time frame. If you feel uncomfortable at any level, cease writing. Otherwise, continue writing until you feel the urge to stop or when your alarm mechanism makes itself known. Then try to analyze what you just wrote.

At times a feeling of drowsiness can occur in automatic writing, but it does not happen to everyone. It is common for the brain to become more easily fatigued when it is not used to holding the energy of the higher octaves. It may be that when you begin to write, your hand and arm will show signs of losing their sensation and any feeling of pain. You may be quite unconscious of this fact and only discover it by accident. Sometimes the message begins at the right-hand side of the page and moves toward the left, like Hebrew. When this is the case, it is a good plan to hold the sheet of paper up to a mirror to see whether the writing can be read in this way. If so, the writing has been reversed and is what is termed "mirror writing."

When finished, thank your guides, teachers, angels of 100% pure Light, and your Higher Self, if appropriate. Then perform a grounding method such as imagining dropping cables from your hip bones and tailbone into the core of the Earth and attaching to the bedrock. Rub your hands briskly together and then hold them with your palms on your face for a few seconds for a quick rejuvenation. Now you can continue with your day.

Automatic Writing Technique: Summary

1. Turn off your phone and remove any other distractions.
2. Gather your notebook and pen. Set your timer.
3. Close your eyes and take three very deep breaths.
4. Acquire a deep and relaxed state of mind, or use alternate nostril breathing, as instructed in Chapter 11, "The Empowerment of Meditation."
5. Request that your Higher Self take full command of you or ask to be connected only with angels, guides, and teachers of 100% pure Light.
6. Think about your intentions for the session.
7. Rest your hand and pen upon the notebook in a writing position.
8. When you notice or feel a connection via colors, warmth, or an elevated mood, state your intentions or pose your question mentally, or say it out loud.

9. With your eyes still closed and your focus on your connection, allow your hand to write what you intuit is the response to your inquiry. Continue writing what you are hearing, seeing, sensing, or knowing without viewing what you are writing as the response.

10. When you are finished writing, or the allotted time is over, express gratitude to the source of information received.

11. Slowly open your eyes. Briskly rub your hands together and place them on your eyes or face for a few moments.

12. End with a Grounding technique of some type (see Chapter 9).

Spiritual Beings of higher vibrations radiate only love, acceptance, and Light. They are present only for the purpose of service to you. They never demand anything of you, and they leave you feeling confident, empowered, and loved. The information they share with you expands your basic knowledge and often enhances your life. The advice they impart allows you freedom to exercise your free will. These true spiritual guides will convey a service of humility, sincerity, and simplicity.

On the other hand, negative entities tend to create confusion, stress, and discomfort. Interaction with these Beings will often be unclear and may even be contradictory to information previously shared with you by your true guides and teachers. You may have a physical or emotional reaction to what they convey to you. Instead of feeling positive and uplifted by their presence, you may feel exhausted. Be on guard for any information that is flattering or attempts to inflate your ego. Be especially aware of being told "you are a chosen one" or that you have been singled out for a certain mission that only you can fulfill. The strength of the negativity of these Beings may produce dread, fear, or anxiety. Other indications of dark-force energy include, but are not limited to, the following:

- A sense of disempowerment
- A sudden onset of health problems
- Sleep disturbances or nightmares
- Longstanding difficulty coping with stress

- Onset of relationship problems
- Frequent mood swings
- Obsession with personal gain and material possessions
- A series of "bad luck" situations
- Increase in personal accidents
- Profound fatigue, especially before spiritual work

The Importance of Discernment

History has revealed that there is a duality established in the universe, back to the beginning of time. This explains the presence of the lower-density, fear-based, evil, and malevolent types of energies also residing on the Earth plane. At this present juncture of the Earth's planned ascension, it is extremely important to help this negative energy be requalified by sending it back to the Light. The various forms of this intense negativity have different attributes. The higher the source of this negativity, the more cunning are the energy characteristics. One of the most common is the ability to disguise this negative energy, albeit for just a short time, and to present a form as coming from the Light. It would be as if they were wearing a Halloween costume of sorts; however, they are unable to sustain this façade for any length of time. In other words, "spiritual" Beings are not always what they say they are or what they appear to be.

Along these lines, not all metaphysical gatherings are solely spiritual ones. Often they are infiltrated by higher-level negative Beings that are there to dissuade seekers from their spiritual path. Thus, the individual who attends metaphysical functions must be wary of unsolicited hugs from strangers. If unsure about hugging another, it is best to focus on your heart center. Then ask mentally if it is for your highest and greatest good to give or receive an embrace. Trust and follow whatever answer is given to you. This is known as *discernment*. Remember, when hugging another, you are entering his or her energy field and blending it with your own. You are also connecting your heart center with someone else, and that may not be for your greatest good. If you do experience an unexpected hug from someone you don't know, immediately call upon Archangel Michael to disconnect you from the other.

While developing discernment is a necessary skill to be cultivated by the seeker, it is even more important to qualify the true source of your daily spiritual guidance. This can be accomplished by means of a simple question: *"Are you of 100% pure Light?"* Then pause a few seconds and wait for an answer. Even if the answer is "yes," state this command three times: *"If you are not of the Light, I command you to leave and cease to exist!"* The negative influence must then depart, according to Universal Law. In addition, it is good to remember that negative energies are not always truthful. So it's helpful to use your body as a barometer.

Since many negative levels of energy from other realms have developed the ability to camouflage their energy as though from the Light, it would be fitting to discuss ways to differentiate them from true guides. Whenever you become aware of the presence of an unfamiliar energy while in a meditative state, immediately tune into its vibration and how your physical body feels. If you should detect any negativity, fear, doubt, apprehension, or resistance, *immediately* command the presence to leave using the Universal Command: *"If you are not of the Light, you must leave now!"* State this command aloud, *forcefully,* three times.

It is also important to implement protection techniques at the start of every meditation session, and upon arising and before falling asleep. This brief process cannot be overemphasized. Besides invading your sleep state, negative entities often appear whenever you are emotionally out of sync, excessively worried, confused, physically depleted, ill, or struggling with an emotionally charged situation. If you should detect any negativity, fear, doubt, anxiety, or resistance, automatically command the presence to disappear and cease to exist. When in doubt, exercise your free will and demand that the energy exit immediately! If it is a true guide, it will remain.

Dream Dynamics

Dreams are tools that serve us in many ways. They give us real experiences of the spiritual world. At the same time, they give us a picture of the current conditions existing in our waking life. They not only provide lessons for us, but they also often assist us in finding a solution to a problem. They can even give us a glimpse of the possible future. Interestingly, many dreams will have more than one function.

Dreams have a characteristic structure that is analogous to a stage play. They always have a theme, which we categorize into a title of some sort for recollection purposes. They always have an opening scene, and are always filled with literal references and symbolism. This symbolism is divided into universal symbols and personal symbols. The universal symbols are those that are common to anyone and would mean the same to all. Examples of this would be stairs or bridges. On the other hand, personal symbols only mean something of significance to the dreamer. This is why it is commonly agreed that the dreamer is the best interpreter of his/ her own dreams. Also, what someone experienced on the day before the dream often influences the choice of symbol used to express a given idea.

People in one's life are frequently used by the dream mind, both as literal representations and as symbols. In actuality, a symbol in a dream is the best possible representation of a very complex and abstract fact that is not yet grasped by the conscious mind.

In order to establish a dream theme or title, there are three basic models to follow. The first one is that someone is doing something to someone. The second model is that someone is in a certain kind of situation. The last model is that things are happening in a certain way. Key themes occur in almost everyone's dreams. Some of the most common dream images include: falling (helplessness, danger, or loss of control); being naked (shame or vulnerability); being chased (guilt or victimization); wild animals (aggression or power); teeth falling out (embarrassment, passivity, or aging); rape (low self-esteem or manipulation); failing an exam (being tested or fear); and paralysis (conflict or an impasse). Dreams often use repetition to draw attention to psychological conflict or an obstacle in someone's life. Dreams repeat motifs to emphasize a point. The repetition may be a single dream, in several dreams in one night, or in dreams over a period of days, months, and even years.

Dreams require a very delicate type of recall. It's a special skill, but it can be easily developed. Perhaps the most effective tool in dream recall is the power of suggestion. This is a way of preprogramming the brain prior to going to sleep. To do this, quietly repeat the following phrase to yourself several times before dozing off. *"Tonight I will remember my dreams."* Another option is to repeat to yourself: *"I will sleep soundly, awaken refreshed, and remember and understand my dreams."* Then arrange a time when you can spontaneously awaken. Prior to sleep, ask to remember what needs to be remembered in your night's adventures and to learn what you need to learn.

The best time to start developing the skill of dream recall is in the morning, after a natural awakening. That's because when you do wake up naturally, without any alarm or voices to jar you, you are more apt to recall aspects of your dream state. Upon awakening, notice how you are feeling. Do you feel nervous or fearful? If you do recall a dream, try to identify the theme or issue of it by reflecting upon whether it is mirroring anything that is currently happening in your life. Since your dream state can help you discover your underlying feelings as well as problem-solving options, be aware of solutions to specific situations that might be revealed to you in your dreams.

Upon awakening, simply lie with your eyes closed, so that visual stimuli will not erase the delicate images still lingering in your mind. If you hit a block, just let your mind wander back to what you were thinking about when you first awoke. One theory is that the dream is best remembered when it is recalled in the position in which it was dreamed. Always try to record your dreams when they are fresh in your memory. That time frame is approximately ten minutes or fewer to catch a dream. After that period, only remnants remain. Perhaps you wish to share a dream experience with a friend whenever possible. Still, be sure to record it as well. In this manner, you'll have a book of knowledge about yourself that will be a treasure for years to come.

Dreams, like all spiritual information shared with you, can become an integral source of your guidance if you will simply develop this vast resource.

Chapter 11

The Empowerment of Meditation

Meditation is the act of listening to Source. It is a state of relaxed concentration, enhanced awareness, and an inward glimpse to the functioning of your mind. Meditation is a skill, and the benefits come with practice and patience. It releases energetic blocks so that energy can flow more effectively throughout the body.

Have you always wondered about meditation but didn't know how to go about learning how to do it? Those who regularly meditate say you can't know the calming effect it brings until you try it. Meditation is free and easy. It can be done practically anywhere since there's no special equipment required. All you need is a quiet place, a commitment to focus, and an open mind.

Meditation is like peeling an onion. There are multiple layers. When one layer is peeled away, the next layer is revealed, and on and on. When beginning, it is best to start with five- to ten-minute sessions. Since I have received so many benefits from meditation, this chapter is devoted entirely to this subject.

Practically every culture has encouraged the practice of some internal focusing techniques. Different names have been given to these various practices of acquiring inner silence. The particular method used to reach inner silence isn't important to the results. True meditation can only begin when you are able to concentrate your consciousness without distractions. Being able to concentrate the mind allows you to direct energy where and when you want it. The daily practice of meditation will not only assist you to unwind from the day's stresses, but can also calm and energize you for the challenges that lie ahead. Some people choose to meditate in the dark before bedtime because it helps them better sleep through the night. Others prefer to start their day meditating, and some choose to meditate daily at both times.

The popularity of meditation is the promise of becoming more relaxed most of the time. It appears to relax the body and offer the mind the opportunity to gain a new perspective. Meditation also trains the capacity to pay attention and thus increases concentration and empathy. This differentiates it from other methods of relaxation, most of which allow the mind to wander wherever it will. This sharpening of attention lasts beyond the meditation session itself. It appears in a variety of ways in the rest of the day. It enhances an individual's ability to notice subtle perceptual cues in the environment and to focus more on the present moment rather than letting the mind wander elsewhere. Other benefits of establishing a consistent daily meditative practice include: changes in breath rate and heart rate; reduction in time urgency; release of physical tensions; and a sudden realization that you did not have any thoughts.

Preparation for Meditation

Identify a quiet place and time. It is helpful to have the security of knowing you will not be interrupted and that your time is your own. Perhaps you are fortunate enough to have someone who will support you and give you the space and time you will need. Find a comfortable chair that allows you to sit upright, or settle yourself into a cross-legged position on the floor. Maintaining good posture with your back straight facilitates attentiveness. It is not a good idea to lie down or become so comfortable that you'll fall asleep. If you are super-tense, roll your neck or shrug your shoulders a few times before beginning. When you are ready, close your eyes. Placing your tongue on the roof of your mouth (just behind the upper teeth) helps to keep your focus. Let your hands rest easily in your lap, palms turned upward in a gesture of receptivity, or close your index fingers and thumbs to form an "O" shape with each hand.

Take three deep breaths. Then continue with deep breaths and count "one" on the inhale, "two" on the exhale, "three" on the inhale, and so on up to the count of ten. Then begin again at "one" when you inhale. If your mind should wander and you forget to count, do not become angry with yourself. After all, you are developing a skill. Just start again. Counting for each breath and dismissing distractions is all you need to do. Think of each distraction as merely an opportunity for more practice. Your breathing will slow, and relaxation will automatically occur. Continue this process until the allotted time is completed, and come out of the meditative state easily by slowly counting from ten to one. Then open your eyes. The first few times you meditate, just spend about five minutes. At your own speed, you will gradually increase to additional time. Each meditation session will be different, so enjoy each one for its unique qualities. I always choose to keep a spiral notebook handy to jot down any revelations that might spring forth organically during my session.

There is not just one way to meditate. Here, again, intention is everything. There is also not just one way to receive messages from the higher realms. You may receive messages in the form of words, music, symbols, colors, sensations, or visualizations seen through your third eye. Each person may receive insights according to the method that is the most prominent way he or she accesses information and via the strongest route that has been developed thus far in his or her spiritual evolution. As stated earlier in this book, there is tremendous support now on the Earth plane for receiving guidance from your spiritual teachers, angels, and guides due to the accelerated vibrations of Mother Earth herself. You just need to pay attention.

Sample Meditations

The Centering Meditation

The Centering Meditation is the most basic and will quickly relax the body, feelings, and thoughts. You may even want to do it first, before practicing any of the other types of meditation. To begin, sit upright in a comfortable position with your spine supported. Close your eyes and relax your body, starting with feet and legs and progressing up your body to your arms, neck, face, and scalp. Relax the muscles behind your eyes as well. Next take a deep breath and release a deep sigh to let go of any pent-up tensions. Allow your mind to become still.

Imagine a point between your eyebrows inside your forehead. At this point, focus all your attention. If thoughts enter, just let them pass through and return your attention to the point of concentration every time the mind wanders. Practice this for a few minutes. Now notice if you can feel your heart beating. Be aware of the rhythm of your breath. Soon a peaceful feeling of being centered within will occur. Your heart and head will seemingly blend as one and melt into a deep center. It is here that you will be able to receive a fresh supply of energy and awareness.

The Breath Meditation

The Breath Meditation is one of the simplest and most widespread of methods, found in almost every ancient spiritual tradition in one form or another. In order to practice this technique, you'll need to find a quiet place in your home where you can be undisturbed. Then turn off your phone. Create a time and place that is yours. Next, get comfortable but not too comfortable. You want to avoid falling asleep. Loosen your belt and any tight clothing. However, you don't have to sit in a yoga position to meditate. A straight-back chair will do fine or anywhere you can sit comfortably while your back is supported. Sit up straight, but relax. Keep your head, neck, and spine aligned as though a large helium balloon were lifting your head upward. Keeping your head upright will help your mind stay more alert. Close your eyes and keep them closed until the session is ended.

Start by bringing your awareness to your breathing, to the natural flow of your breath as it comes and goes through your nostrils. Don't follow your breath in your body or out into the air. Just be aware as it comes and goes through your nostrils. Be sensitive to actual sensations of your breath ... to the movement or air ... to its warmth ... to however you feel. Don't try to control your breath; just be aware of it as you breathe in and out. If your breath becomes more shallow, let it be shallow. If it gets faster or slower, let it. The breath regulates itself. While you meditate, your job is simply to be aware of it. Whenever you notice that your mind has wandered, gently return it to your breath.

During the meditation, you tell yourself that everything other than your breath—such as thoughts, plans, memories, sounds, and sensations—are distractions. Let go of your other thoughts. Whatever comes into your mind besides your breath is now a distraction. Don't blame yourself if your mind wanders. It's only natural. Just gently bring your focus back to your breath each time. To help keep your mind fixed on your breath, you can silently label each inhalation as "one" and each exhalation as "two." Stay in touch, though, with the actual experience of breathing, not merely the repetition of the words and numbers. Let your breath come and go at its natural rhythm.

When you are ready to stop, take a moment just to be with your body. Notice how you feel. Then open your eyes.

To obtain maximum results from this meditation, try to practice daily for ten to fifteen minutes. If you want, you can gradually extend your meditation to about half an hour. You may wish to add music.

Body-Scan Meditation

In this meditation, you merely move your mind through your body. By mentally allowing each area to relax fully, you can reach a deep state of physical relaxation. This particular meditation can be done either sitting or lying down on your back. The first thing to do is to eliminate anything that would agitate your mind in any manner.

Start by bringing your attention to the forehead area. Be aware of any sensations that are present. Pay particular attention to the muscle that creates a frown, just above the nose. If there is any tension there, let the muscle soften and relax.

Scan each eyebrow and eye area. Relax all the tiny muscles around and behind each eye. Continue to scan your facial muscles from side to side. If you notice any tension, allow it to soften or melt away. Next scan each ear and relax any tension in the scalp. Scan from above the forehead down to the back of your neck, going from side to side.

Then all around your neck, scan from the throat around each side to the spine at the back. Continue letting all the tense muscles soften and relax. Now scan each shoulder down to the elbow and the hand. Continue with a side-to-side scanning. Relax any tension.

Now move to the top of the back and beneath the neck. Begin to scan down your spine and from side to side. Let the muscles in your shoulder blades and upper and lower back become loose and limp.

Move down into your pelvis area and release any tension located there. Move down into each leg and foot as you scan side to side and let go of any muscular tensions.

With your mind, now freely scan through your entire body. Wherever you find any remaining tension, let the muscles soften and relax. When you are ready to stop, open your eyes and carry this calm peacefulness with you throughout the remainder of the day.

Walking Meditation

This meditation is particularly useful for people who find it difficult to sit still while they meditate or have difficulty focusing their mind. In walking meditation, you make all the minuscule sensations of walking the focus of the meditation. This gives your mind more to notice than just the breath and makes concentration easier. It is important to find a quiet place where you can walk undisturbed and undistracted. All you need is a clear area where you can walk a minimum of eight to ten steps and then reverse. The point is not to walk anywhere in particular, but to pay attention to the act of walking.

Begin by standing with your feet shoulder width apart. Allow your arms to hang comfortably at your sides. Slowly shift your weight back and forth on each foot. Notice the changes and sensations of movement, tension, and pressure. Begin to extend your left foot slowly forward and take a slow and deliberate step. As you move, be fully aware of the sensations of your entire leg and foot. Pay attention to everything you can experience in the process of walking; however, do not watch your legs as you walk. Just sense them. Keep your eyes softly focused on the path ahead of you. When you reach the end of your path, stop and turn with full awareness of the nuances of the movement.

As you continue walking back and forth, you can assist your mind's focus by silently stating "lifting" as you lift the leg, "moving" as you move forward, and "placing" as you lower the leg. If your mind wanders, gently return it to the sensations in your legs and feet. When it is time to stop, become aware of the sensations in all your extremities as well as your entire body. Carry this focused calm to whatever you do next.

Protective Meditation

Sometimes people will see a frightening image while meditating, like they do in dreams and nightmares. However, in meditation unlike a nightmare, you are conscious and can always change your consciousness. You need to understand that you can protect yourself from yourself. Evil images are part of your own consciousness, just as angels are of your consciousness also. When anything scary starts to occur, you can quickly use your will to say, *"I AM the master of myself,"* and tell the intruder to leave your meditation. Then you can mentally wash away all fear and negative energy by visualizing the color pink, and replacing negativity with love and Light. Unfortunately, sometimes people can zap you with bad energy. You can protect yourself with the following meditation.

Close your eyes, take three deep breaths, quiet your mind, and become still. Dismiss all extraneous thoughts and replace them with thoughts of peace and harmony. Then imagine a beautiful shimmering White Light coming from the top of your head like a gushing waterfall, filling your entire body. Feel the White Light flow into your face, your eyes, ears, nose, and mouth. Feel it pour down into your neck, chest, arms, and into your hands. Next imagine it filling up your heart center with peaceful, blissful White Light. Feel it as it flows into your stomach, down through your buttocks, into your thighs, knees, calves, feet, and out through your toes. Imagine yourself turning into a pure white waterfall. Become aware of the freshness of the energy as it gushes in, out, and all around you. Feel it cleansing you of any fearful thoughts or negative feelings. Feel it protect you like a shield of brilliant soothing Light. Allow this Light to permeate every cell of your body. Stay in this peacefulness for a while, and then gradually emerge from this meditative state.

Pranayama Yoga Technique

This very ancient breathing technique helps to balance both hemispheres of your brain, your subtle bodies, your nervous system, and the right and left sides of your body. When you first begin this type of specific yogic breathing, you may notice at times that it is easier to breathe through one nostril than through the other. This is a normal occurrence.

You can use the thumb of your right hand to close your right nostril and then switch to use the ring finger of the right hand to close the left nostril. Start by closing the right nostril and fully inhale through the left nostril. Then close the left nostril and exhale fully through the right nostril. Now inhale through the right nostril as the left remains closed. Finally, exhale through the left nostril (the right one is closed). Repeat this series, alternating nostrils after each inhalation.

Following is another version of alternate nostril breathing that I learned from my meditation teacher, Raj.

Alternate Nostril Breathing

In 1987 I began my practice of meditation to assist me with coping with a highly stressful management job while also attending graduate school. I took meditation lessons twice a week for four years. My meditation teacher was Rajendra (Raj) Khanna, who was the proprietor of a small Eastern Indian artifact store in downtown Cleveland, Ohio. Raj was a journalist, poet, linguist, lecturer, and teacher of both yoga and meditation. He migrated to the United States from India in 1974 at the age of sixty-one and settled in the Cleveland area, where three of his children lived. He was seventy-three years old when I first met him, and he could still perform many of the yoga asanas. He quickly became a major catalyst for my spiritual development.

Many of my insights about life, as well as creative endeavors, have sprung forth from my meditation practice. These daily sessions helped me keep everything in perspective, which was something my conscious mind was unable to do. Meditation instilled calmness within me that I could access at any moment of my choosing. This process is very difficult unless there is a frame of reference about what relaxation feels like to you. By adopting a meditative practice, I was able to heal my body, calm my mind, and de-stress my life. Daily meditation has been the most significant factor in my spiritual evolution on multiple levels.

According to Raj, the quest for peace and happiness lies deep in everyone's heart. Most seek them outside, in external things. However, real peace and real happiness come from within. This requires a change of focus, a change in attitude, and a change from the physical consciousness to the inner or higher consciousness. He emphasized that a pure mind and a pure heart will create a pure body.

The method of meditation he espoused was one of alternate nostril breathing. This is an important basic yoga technique. Using this technique helps to integrate the left and right sides of the brain, establishing a sense of calmness. The sequence of breathing was done in three to five cycles. After that, I was to focus on the present moment and allow all thoughts just to drift by without dwelling upon them. For the full benefit of meditation to arise, it must be practiced consistently on a daily basis, even if only for ten minutes at a time. It is important to wear clean, loose clothing. It is better to do any spiritual work before eating to allow the body to support the spiritual experience fully rather than be overwhelmed with processing a meal. At the end of each meditation session is a good time to choose to send love and good wishes to anyone who might have caused negativity in your life. I was also encouraged to keep a journal of what transpired during my meditation sessions, as insights will often be discovered during the process. Frequently these insights were from past-life recalls.

I started with ten minutes daily of meditation following the breathing rounds. Raj instructed me to face eastward when I meditated in the morning and then I could draw energy to me from the sun. If I meditated at night, I was to face north so I could draw energy from the Earth due to the magnetic force of the North Pole. Soon I meditated for twenty minutes twice a day and noticed that I slept more soundly at night. Eventually (over several years' time) I progressed to forty-five minutes daily. When meditation is consistently practiced at the same time daily, it allows the angels and guides to connect with us and share their wisdom since the usual mind chatter has been erased.

Alternate Nostril Breathing Technique

The following technique allows you to inhale through one nostril and exhale out the other in a specific manner of inhalation, holding, and then exhalation. This pattern is then reversed for a complete round of breathing. After obtaining a comfortable meditation posture with your back straight, the exact process of this particular form of rhythmic breathing is as follows:

1. Close your eyes. Then with either hand, use your fingers to close the right nostril.
2. Slowly inhale a complete breath through the left nostril for four counts. (The count is to the rate of a sweeping second hand on a watch or clock.)
3. Hold the breath, closing both nostrils to the count of sixteen.
4. Slowly exhale through the right nostril, keeping the left nostril closed, counting to eight.
5. Close both nostrils again and count to four.
6. Now reverse the process.
7. Keeping the right nostril open (the left nostril is closed), slowly inhale the total breath for four counts.
8. Hold the breath, closing both nostrils to the count of sixteen.

9. Then breathe out through the left nostril, with the right nostril closed, for the count of eight.

10. Close both nostrils again and count to four.

This is the completion of one full cycle, or round, out of three to five rounds total.

Repeat this sequence with the left nostril, as before, then with the right nostril, and finally with the left nostril again. Thus you will be doing this 4, 16, 8, and 4 rhythmic breathing three to five times in all, with alternating nostrils. Continue the breath by alternating the nostrils as above, until you have completed the desired number of rounds. When you are finished with the sequence, take a few deep breaths to return your breathing to normal. After finishing these breathing cycles, you will feel calm waves of energy flowing through your entire body. The first few times you practice the breath, you may feel slightly dizzy or light-headed. This might happen because your body is not accustomed to the increased oxygen to the brain. Always keep your tongue on the roof of your mouth to help keep your focus. This connects two master meridians, the Conception Vessel that travels up the front of the body and ends at the tip of the tongue, and the Governing Vessel that travels up the back of the body and ends at the roof of the mouth.

Now in your mind's eye, select something that has significance to you. This will become your Focal Point for all meditation practices. Excluding humans, it can be a tree, flower, scene, lighted candle, or an image of a spiritual figure. Once your choice is made, you will concentrate on this Focal Point for ten minutes as you hold the image by visualization or intention. Continue to focus exclusively on this mental vision. It is not as easy as it sounds, as our minds are not often trained for this discipline. In addition, two to five times a day, focus on the Focal Point for several short periods of time.

During this concentration process, many thoughts will enter your mind. The goal of meditation is to not interact with any of them. Acknowledge each thought, and then brush it aside as you return your concentration to your Focal Point. Mentally say: *"I see you* [the thought]. *Now please go away so I can meditate."* Then brush aside any thoughts and keep returning to the Focal Point. Meditation cannot be forced. Meditation happens. Continue this process repeatedly as you train your mind to hold only one thought—that of your Focal Point. Thinking about something else while in meditation can be brought about for various reasons such as fears, sleeplessness, noises, pain, and body restlessness. To overcome your mind wandering, you can form a habit of recall. Fix your mind on the Focal Point and bring your attention back to that point whenever it wanders from it. The habit of recall will eventually replace the habit of wandering and will bring the object of concentration back to the central point.

After a few weeks of diligence on a daily basis, you will be able to concentrate on your preselected image much more easily. Whenever the Focal Point disappears, mentally retrieve it. Continue this process again, and again, and again. In time, you will be able to hold the Focal Point for longer durations, and the number of extraneous thoughts will decrease. Eventually you will begin drifting toward actual meditational states and higher levels of awareness. Allow approximately one half hour for six to eight months, then you can slowly extend the time as you desire. Do not be alarmed by your imagination during your meditations, as it is this aspect of you that is creating your future. Allow yourself to be open to the beauty of the unseen world through the support of your creativity and imagination. The key for this to unfold perfectly is always to align your thoughts, desires, and goals for your highest and greatest good.

Often during meditation the sense of timing is altered, so it is a good idea to utilize a chime, an alarm, or a timer to enable you to adhere to the allocated time frame. You can also purchase meditation alarms that have soothing bells or chimes. Once the timer device is set, it is easier to relax and forget about the time. Due to modern technology, I even have a meditation timer application on my phone. When you hear the alarm sound, slowly and gently open your eyes and blink a few times. Rub your palms briskly together and place them over both eyes. Move your body and bring it back to a normal state of awareness. Ground yourself, if needed. Then drink some water. I strongly recommend that you end each meditation session by recording what you experienced. Don't wait until later on in your day, or the next day, to do this. When you are meditating, you are not in a normal waking state of consciousness. Like a dream, the awarenesses gleaned in your meditative state can slip away within ten minutes. Days or weeks later, when you read what you wrote, you will naturally have forgotten some of it. You may even choose to keep your meditation recordings in a special notebook.

After three or four months of practice, the breathing rhythm can be increased to 6-24-12-6. Then a few months later, it can be increased to 8-32-16-8. Within a year, if a person has been meditating daily, the breathing rhythm can be increased to 10-40-20-10. However, it is important to note that if the accelerated level creates any discomfort, you must return to the previous level until a future time.

At times, as an individual progresses with an accelerated meditation practice, certain "Divine Sounds" may be evident as the person reaches another vibrational level. These may include:

- Buzzing of bees sound
- Waves dashing against the rocks sound
- Sound of a flute
- Wind passing through a cluster of bushes sound
- Om sound

Breathing Sequences

First 3 weeks:	4-16-8-4	Do 3 to 5 cycles
After 3 weeks:	6-24-12-6	Do 4 or 5 cycles
After 6 weeks:	8-32-16-8	
Then:	10-40-20-10	
Next:	12-48-24-12	
Continue:	14-56-28-14	
Progress:	16-64-32-16	
Then:	18-72-36-18	
Next:	20-80-40-20	

Continue: 24-96-48-24
Progress: 30-120-60-30

Establishing Protection for Your Meditations

It is paramount prior to any type of meditation that you protect your auric field. This can be accomplished by creating a strong protective shield or bubble around you or White Light as a force field. You can either visualize its existence surrounding you, or you can simply state the intention for its creation aloud. The White Light is always available for your daily protection, including at the beginning of your meditations, by simply stating the intention that it be established and that it completely surround you with a protective shield. Other techniques for protection are found throughout this book, particularly Chapters 5, 6, and 7.

Even though the White Light is invisible to the eye, do not underestimate the power of its protection. Although there are many examples, I'll recall here one situation that can demonstrate the effectiveness of this force field of White Light. One afternoon after leaving my meditation session to go to my grad school class in downtown Cleveland, Ohio, I suddenly noticed that I was being followed to my car in a parking lot by three thug-looking teenagers. Since this was in an area where there had been frequent purse snatchings, I was on high alert. I started visualizing the White Light totally encasing me as I walked to my car, holding my purse close to my body. My car key was in a position to protect myself. They walked right up to my car as I jumped in and closed the door. Then they all looked at me as they nonchalantly walked past.

As for grounding techniques, there are many variations, but most have you imagine a connection with the Earth. (See Chapter 9 for several Grounding techniques.) This can occur by visualizing cables dropping from your tailbone and hip bones to deep within the core of the Earth. Then visualize the cables adhering to the Earth's bedrock as you breathe in deep nurturing, grounding Earth energy up from the cables into your physical body. You can also imagine dropping an anchor, rope, or taproot from a tree and reaching down deep within the Earth. Your physical body will feel safe when you imagine this grounding connection to the Earth as part of your meditation process. Physically you can also ground yourself by hugging an old tree, walking barefoot, sitting on the ground, or holding specific stones such as hematite, obsidian, or amber. If you are going to be in environments where there is much tension, conflict, or anger, it's best to keep black obsidian or black tourmaline in your pocket. If you carry these stones daily, they need to be rinsed under running water each day to wash away the negative energies they have absorbed.

No matter how long you meditate, remember that if you don't find the time daily, doing it at least occasionally is better than not at all. Don't yield so easily to the temptation to do something that suddenly seems more urgent or useful. When you are able to dismiss all extraneous thoughts and replace them with thoughts of peace and harmony, then you can experience the joyful process of discovery that meditation creates. By entering into the secret recesses of your inner being, you can come into contact with your True Self. No one can bring you into contact with your True Self except you. You may be shown or told what to do, but you must take the necessary steps alone. The best method to use is meditation.

Balance Meditation

Allow yourself to become comfortable in a place where you will not be disturbed. Gently close your eyes. Take a deep breath and mentally hold it to the count of four. Now exhale slowly as you mentally count backward from eight to one. Then take two more deep breaths in the same manner.

In your mind's eye create a relaxing scene somewhere out in nature. Visualize it utilizing all your senses. Now imagine a beautiful ray of sunshine beaming down into your body at the base of your spine and forming a bubble of energy around your root chakra. Allow this beam of sunshine to harmonize and balance this first chakra. Say the word "Balance" verbally. Then ask the Universe for the correct color of red to be anchored there, allowing your vibrations to increase.

When that feels complete, notice that the beam of sunshine moves up to your second chakra and forms a bubble of energy around your spleen area. Imagine this ray of sunshine harmonizing and balancing the energies of your second chakra. Say the word "Balance" verbally. Then ask the Universe for the correct color of orange to be anchored there, vitalizing your life-force energy.

The sunlight beam now moves up to form a bubble of energy over your solar plexus chakra to heal, balance, and harmonize your third chakra. Say the word "Balance" verbally. Anchor and visualize the color yellow in this chakra and become aware of your personal power as the sunlight energy vibrates and harmonizes this power center. When this area feels balanced, notice that the beam of vibrant sun energy continues moving up to your heart center.

This bright sun energy now forms a bubble over your fourth chakra, and as it vibrates, it balances and harmonizes the energies of your heart chakra. Say the word "Balance" verbally. Focus your awareness on your heart and feel it becoming warmer. Notice that you can radiate energy out from your heart to others in waves. Ask the Universe to anchor the correct color of green into this chakra and feel the love that is sent to you from the Universe.

The beam of sunlight continues to move upward to your throat area. Notice that a bubble of sunshine has formed over your throat chakra. Allow this bubble to harmonize and balance the energies in your fifth chakra. Verbally say the word "Balance." Ask the Universe to anchor the color of blue in this area to increase your spiritual awareness.

The sunlight now moves up to your brow area and forms a bubble over your third eye. As the bubble of sun energy vibrates, it activates your spiritual vision while balancing and harmonizing the energy in your sixth chakra. Say the word "Balance" verbally. Ask the Universe to anchor the color indigo in this area and bathe you in wisdom. When this feels complete, notice that the ray of sunlight moves to the top of your head.

Now a protective bubble of sunlight energy is formed over your crown chakra, and this area is balanced and harmonized. Verbally say the word "Balance." Allow this energy to activate the powers of your mind and spirit. Ask the Universe to anchor the color violet in this area as you reestablish your connection to Source. When this connection has occurred, allow the beam of sunshine to radiate and vitalize each chakra and then spew out the top of your head, cascading down around your body like a waterfall. When you are ready, count mentally from one to ten. Slowly open your eyes and revel in this state of balance.

As you can see, there is a variety of techniques to assist you to become focused and centered in a meditative state. The following recommendations may be helpful as you develop your skills at achieving a state of inner silence and peace.

- Avoid any disturbance.
- Be comfortable.
- Limit the time of your meditative sessions.
- Select the right meditative technique for you.
- Do not meditate after eating.
- Disregard distracting thoughts.
- Meditate routinely at the same time of the day.
- Emerge from the meditative state easily and slowly.
- Enjoy each session for its unique qualities.
- Keep a journal of your experiences.
- Continued practice leads to cumulative benefits.
- Avoid meditation when you are tired.
- Practice, practice, practice.

Chapter 12

Toward Energy Mastery

Everything you can see, hear, feel, smell, or taste is a form of energy, all vibrating at different rates. Scientists are in agreement that all physical matter is composed of atoms. These atoms are made from electrons, protons, and neutrons, all in perpetual motion and moving at incredibly high speeds.[1] Energy extends far beyond the Earth plane to the atmosphere and the space beyond the Earth and our solar system to the distant stars and planets of the Universe. All is one large mass of vibrating energy. You are surrounded by energy even though you may not see it. Everything you perceive is energy, whether visible or invisible, audible or inaudible. For instance, you cannot visually see air, electricity, or sound, yet each has a profound effect on your physical body function. Although these energies are not visible, they can be perceived though the vibrations we experience via our aura.

The energy field surrounding your physical body merges with your physical nervous system. When you come in contact with other energies, either positive or negative, your brain picks up the sensation through signals from the nervous system. The experience is then interpreted, an impression is made, and an action is initiated. The aura is a bio-energetic component of you. It is depicted as having several separate sheaths or layers that ultimately combine to form the whole. It includes your feelings, emotions, vibrations, and level of vitality. Thus humans are permeated with life-force energy vibrating at different rates. The molecular composition of the physical body is a complex matrix of interwoven energy fields.[2]

Emotional Release

As I stated previously, thoughts and feelings are not always ours. We walk through thought-forms all day long. Some even linger at ancient sites or places where large throngs of people frequent. So, how do you know if the emotions you are experiencing actually belong to you? The most accurate way is to place your dominant hand on your chest and tune into your heart as you ask: *"Does this belong to me?"* Then it is very important to trust the immediate first response that you receive. If it is yours you can use the Emotional Freedom Technique (EFT) to release it. However, if it does *not* belong to you, the following technique will be very useful for you to release it.

Start by identifying the predominant emotion that you are experiencing. Be precise. Do not use general terms such as "feeling bad." Once the emotional state is identified, say the following: *"I do not accept this [insert the emotion]. I send it back to the sender one thousand fold with divine love!"* State this phrase three times *with emphasis* on each emotion that you are feeling. Often, one emotion can overlay another. An example is sending anxiety or fear away and then feeling confused or angry.

Releasing Cords and Attachments

Often individuals who are depleted of life force unconsciously connect with people who have more life-force energy and siphon off that energy to support their own depleted system. Any emotional exchange between two people creates a flow of astral energies. A cord, as referred to here, is like an etheric astral pipeline through which energies and emotions continuously circulate, and it is a link to someone else's consciousness. All cords are generated by the two people they link and are created by an intense emotional association. Individuals can be attached etherically to every person they have ever known, and every single attachment is acting as a type of energetic drain. I recommend that every person sever all cords that are no longer for their Highest Good to every person or place prior to going to bed at night. Since we have a finite amount of energy within our bodies, you cannot afford for people to take your energy without being replenished.[3]

Individuals not only transmit emotional currents to others, they receive life-force energy from others. When a man and a woman live together, their constant emotional interaction is an initial factor that creates a cord between them. Sleeping in the same bed for years adds to that by creating an intermingling of etheric energies. Sexual intercourse is a deep exchange, one in which a lot of life force is involved and both people's auras are merged. Attachments are lines of energy resembling cords or lines of light, which enter into the chakras and connect and attach people to each other. These cords are passed back and forth between people's chakras constantly, often without the people being aware of it occurring.[4]

These energetic attachments allow the energy created from past interactions to flow backward and forward between the two individuals. This process stimulates the individuals to repeat patterns of behaviors. These cords are usually unnecessary clutter and potential energy drains that can become debilitating and stagnant. Often they cause fatigue, depression, codependence, feelings of victimization, burdensome responsibilities, and communication difficulties. These attachments, however, cannot be connected or received unless the individuals are willing to do so physically, emotionally, or spiritually. Frequently, the discovery of these cords leads to a reexamination of the nature of such relationships. Cords can be removed periodically as a maintenance measure, or daily as a routine, or as an emergency technique. If removed on a daily basis, it is best to do it at the end of the day, before going to sleep.

Cords have different meanings and effects in each chakra. Body scanning is a mindfulness meditation technique whereby you can focus your attention on various parts of your body. Similar to progressive muscle relaxation, you begin at your feet and progress your way up your body. However, instead of tensing and relaxing your muscles, you merely focus on the way each part of your body feels. Next, scan each chakra for any blockages and to assess that the correct color ray is anchored in each one.

First Chakra: This is the survival center. A cord into this chakra means "I want you to help me survive."

Second Chakra: This is the center for sexuality and emotion. A cord in this area means "I need you to give me emotional support."

Third Chakra: This is the power center. A cord in this chakra means "I want to operate on your energy instead of my own."

Fourth Chakra: This is the center of love. A cord in this chakra means "I love you." Unfortunately, these cords could be left over from past relationships.

Fifth Chakra: This is the communication center. A cord in this chakra means "I don't want you to say what you want to say."

Sixth Chakra: This is the center for inner vision. A cord in this chakra means "I am thinking of you."

Seventh Chakra: This is the center of intuition. A cord in this chakra means "I want to control you."

The person who is doing the cording may be doing so on an unconscious level. Cords may also be found in your hand and foot chakras, blocking creativity and contributing to a feeling of being ungrounded.[5]

Whenever you sense, visualize, or otherwise become aware of any cords or attachments, immediately call forth Archangel Michael. Ask him to sever all cords and attachments from any person, place, or thing that are not for your highest good. In fact, this is an excellent daily routine to add to your preparations for sleep each night.

Body Elemental

A Body Elemental is assigned to each individual as well as a Ministering Angel (commonly called a Guardian or Solar Angel). These same beings stay with the person through all embodiments.[6]

Before taking our first embodiment on Earth, we were each called before the Karmic Board. In a solemn ceremony, we were each assigned an elemental being, called a "Body Elemental." At this ceremony, the Body Elemental assumed the obligation to stay with us during each successive embodiment until we reach Ascension. The Body Elemental's purposes are:

1. To cooperate with the True Self in the creation of the physical body from the moment of conception to full growth;

2. To perform certain "involuntary functions" of the physical body, such as breathing, digestion, and maintaining a heartbeat.

3. To keep at all times the physical body as well as the etheric, mental, and emotional bodies in a good state of maintenance.

Our Body Elemental is a physical mentor that stays with us until our life terminates. Since it belongs to the Elemental Kingdom, it is in service to humanity. Its work with the physical body is invisible in nature. It resembles the electric current that supplies power to the bulb that lights a room, offering brightness and visibility while the original source remains invisible.[7]

This highly evolved Etheric Elemental has volunteered to work with physical substance in the continual repair of the physical body. In order to heal, an individual must call it forth in love and work with it in cooperation to restore the physical body. It is the Body Elemental on the etheric plane that can view the Divine Blueprint and then work through the nervous system to produce a similar effect in the physical realm. Therefore, it is beneficial that you discover and become familiar with your own Body Elemental. This can be achieved by acknowledging it, loving it, and treating it with gratitude on a daily basis. You can request that your I AM Presence acquaint you with your Body Elemental as you sleep and then bring forth a conscious awakened memory of that experience.

The Body Elemental is part of the natural process of restoration, and for healing to take place, it is important to have its cooperation. The Body Elemental can best of all restore a distorted etheric pattern for an organ and manifest a corresponding physical change. That Elemental is in tune with the different vibratory patterns and habits of each of the various organs and body parts, and with your cooperation can apply that knowledge to healing, whenever it is invoked. Be sure to build this relationship in times of health and vigor as well as dis-ease.[8]

Healing, from the etheric viewpoint, requires cleansing through the use of the Violet Fire, visualizations, and experiences that focus on opening the vital centers and lines of flow. It also requires physical therapies such as manipulation of the nerves and etheric channels, good nutrition, and toning of the body, along with the correct amount of sunshine, natural vitamins, and other sources of vital force.[9]

To contact your Body Elemental, take time to be silent and to breathe. Notice your posture and any areas of discomfort in your body. Take three deep breaths and then take a moment to reflect on your experience of life in a body. Do you need to make healthier lifestyle choices? What would that take on a daily basis? Have you been ignoring messages that your body has been sending you?[10] Does your Body Elemental have a name? What does it wish to be called?

Ask your Body Elemental's cooperation in looking upon your Divine Blueprint of your True Self and restoring your body to that pattern. Speak to it firmly but lovingly, and acknowledge its service. Invoke next the Angels of Violet Fire to transmute the cause of any illness. As it is being done, ask your I AM Presence to illumine your mind as best as possible, in order for you to discern the lesson to be learned in the creation of that illness.

Body Elemental Meditation

Place your attention on your I AM Presence and your Body Elemental. Radiate your love and gratitude to this blessed friend who has been with you during all your former embodiments and who has taken the vow to be with you until your ascension.

Call on the Law of Forgiveness for all the wrong you have done that may have hurt your relationship with the Body Elemental. Now call on the Violet Flame to cleanse your etheric body, to remove the causes, cores, and effects of past wrong thoughts, feelings, and action. (This will give the Body Elemental a perfect pattern to work with.)[11]

How Not to Take Things On

In the course of your spiritual evolution, it is vital that you take responsibility for how you think and feel. Feelings always follow thought and perception. If you don't like how you are feeling, then change what you are thinking. Take a moment to assess your emotional reactions to certain comments or situations. Take any opportunity where emotions erupt to go inward and assess what needs to be released. As you release the underlying (root) causes of the emotion, you will discover that the process raises your vibrations. The result will be that fewer people will push your emotional buttons. You will become more emotionally balanced. Once emotional triggers are released, you will no longer magnetize negative situations to you. Rather than judging yourself when you lose your composure, take it in stride and thank yourself for the opportunity to reveal another option to heal an unresolved issue. This then will ultimately become a strength. Choose to have only positive thoughts about others and yourself. Stay focused on the present and learn to live in each and every moment. Service is the key to Unity Consciousness. Every day do something for someone else for no reason or expectation. Other options are:

- Develop good sleeping habits.
- Incorporate a daily spiritual regimen.
- Release judgments of yourself and others.
- Adhere to a daily fitness regime.
- Avoid sugar, artificial stimulants, drugs, and GMO foods.
- Create a time for play frequently.
- Spend ten to twenty minutes a day outdoors, if possible.
- Drink plenty of water.
- Take vitamin D3 on a daily basis.
- Write in a journal.
- Regularly recite the Cosmic Law of Forgiveness.
- Keep a positive mental outlook.

- Sleep as much as possible for physical rejuvenation.
- Maintain faith.
- Frequently evoke the Violet Fire.
- Allow daily time to experience inner silence.
- Align the four lower bodies by bringing your hand over your head and then moving it vertically down the front of the body to align the mental, emotional, etheric, and physical bodies.
- Surround the self with White Light surrounded by Blue Light.
- Radiate Divine love into the world from your heart each day.
- Observe your thoughts at work, when conversing, or while you are solving a problem. Watch how you behave and think throughout the day.
- Take frequent rest periods and short doses of exercise.
- Juice frequently, eat the rainbow, and make alkaline food choices.
- Cleanse your aura regularly by adding one cup of baking soda, one cup of sea salt, and one cup of apple cider vinegar to a bathtub full of hot water. Then soak in it for twenty to thirty minutes.
- Focus on the breath.
- An alkaline, live, and organic diet is optimum. Eat local produce from local farmers.
- Avoid as much processed food as possible. Bless your food before you eat.
- Purchase and wear clothing with natural fibers like cotton, hemp, and silk.
- Wear or carry crystals and gemstones that enhance your electromagnetic field and raise your vibrations. Certain gemstones are very effective in helping you stay grounded (deeply connected with Mother Earth), centered, and connected to the present moment. This information is discussed more in Chapter 7, the section entitled "Spiritual Stone Power."

- Give thanks before eating, as the gratitude places you in your heart center. Dr. Masaru Emoto and others have demonstrated that positive emotions and thoughts can change the molecular structure of water, and our body is largely composed of water.[12]

- Protect yourself from potentially harmful radiation when using cell phones, computers, and tablets.

- Using essential oils can enhance the immune system and remove toxins. There is more information on essential oils in Chapter 7, "Spiritual Power Tools."

- Listen to your intuition to guide you to the appropriate practitioners for help.

- Avoid skin hunger by receiving regular healthy touch or trading healing modalities with others.

- Develop a support system of like-minded souls. Join a group or a community to share your ideas and experiences.

- Do not take anything personally.

- Reevaluate your friends and acquaintances and surround yourself with positive and supportive people.

- Keep life as simple as you can.

- Pay it forward whenever possible.

- Keep trying things out until you find the thing that works.

- Don't be attached to anything working the way you would have expected it to in the past.

- Be non-judgmental to others and, most of all, yourself. Instead focus on what is right with you.

- Be in nature as much as you are able and plant flowers, herbs, and vegetables, using heirloom seeds whenever you can.

- Consider saying this shorter version of the Cosmic Law of Forgiveness as part of your daily practice.
  I invoke the Cosmic Law of Forgiveness for myself.
  I forgive myself for anything I have done to anyone and
  I forgive anyone for anything they have done to me.
  So be it, So be it, So be it!

Say the above three times emphatically. If there is a specific individual you are thinking about, use his or her name.

Past-Life Regression

Past-life regression is a valuable tool for enhancing the quality of your present life. You are the sum of all your past experiences. Consequently, knowledge of all your past experiences and how they affect your current reactions and relationships can be quite meaningful. This insight can bring you a clearer understanding of your strengths and weaknesses, personal problems, and negative relationships. It can also show you your purpose for this present sojourn.

The regressive experience generates tolerance and understanding of other cultures, races, and the opposite sex. In this way it assists the individual in developing into a balanced and more complete person. It opens the door to the realization of personal responsibility and helps absolve unnecessary and unhealthy guilt feelings. At the same time, this experience allows people to delve into the recesses of their mind and grasp information, values, and comprehension from both a practical and spiritual perspective.

Past-life experiences allow an individual a healthy outlet for the release of anger, anxiety, frustration, and fear, which all contribute to mental, spiritual, and physical dis-ease. With the changes in attitude and life perspective that are generated by the regressive experience, the individual often discovers that there are fewer situations in the future that initiate anger, frustration, and stress. An individual becomes more relaxed and approaches life with a healthier mental and emotional state. This positive thrust ultimately promotes a healthier body. In addition, a change in attitude can be the key that opens the door to success and happiness. With a more positive attitude, people can find something in almost any situation that can be a benefit to them.

There is a multitude of experiences from past lives that can impact your present daily life. Through the years of working with regressions, both my own and facilitating others, I've found that there are few situations which haven't been explored. Examples include the recognition and understanding of fears, phobias, addictions, infertility, obesity, physical illnesses, limiting decisions, intense relationships, gender identity, confusion, and loneliness. Often these explorations serve as a guide to recognize significant and recurring positive and negative patterns. Other revelations that surface are those of prejudices, family frictions, problem relationships, and geographical and historical fascinations.

Past-life regression is tuning into the subconscious to recall memories. Sometimes the experience occurs spontaneously by a precipitating factor that jogs the memory. Meditation is another method by which past-life memories can be recalled or surface into your awareness.

Hypnosis is probably the most frequently used method for past-life regressions. When facilitated by a qualified and experienced hypnotherapist, it is a very effective method to access knowledge of past lifetimes. This knowledge often engenders the courage to understand and address problems that might otherwise be avoided.

Shielding, or protective techniques, should always be applied prior to a past-life regression session. This consists of the person surrounding him- or herself in a thick cocoon of pure White Light as spiritual protection from any negativity that might be encountered during the exploration.

Many people are curious about what they will experience in a past-life regression. An individual may receive information in several ways. Most commonly there is the sensation of being an observer and watching events unfold in a detached manner. Another reaction is appearing "to know" or be aware of the situation without visualizing it. Sometimes the person will get an unfocused quick impression that tends to disappear just as they are about to grasp it.

Interestingly, it is not necessary for a person to believe in the theory of reincarnation for the regressive experience to be valid and valuable. Reliving what seem to be past-life experiences can help people understand why they do what they do, and show them how to avoid repeating mistakes. It allows the individual involved to immediately take responsibility for his or her actions and healing, rather than developing dependence on a therapist.

Eliminating the fear of death is one of the greatest benefits of the regression experience. Death itself is not a traumatic experience. All pain and discomforts are completely removed at the moment of death. The realization that death is a transitional state, and not a state of termination, often brings profound relief to the person.

Past-life regression is not a panacea. It is a tool to help us reshape our present self, erase karma through forgiveness, and assist us in shaping the future. By looking within ourselves, we can improve our individual lives. Past-life regression is one more step on the path to self-awareness. It is truly a fascinating journey.

Chapter 13

Energy Matrix of Chakras

The major points where the etheric body interconnects with the physical body are called the chakra centers. Etherically these centers look like spinning wheels of light and color. Physically they are represented by major collections of nerve cells along the spine, plus an endocrine gland closely linked to that nerve center. Their purpose is to function as the principal organizing and coordination center of energy flow in both the etheric and physical bodies.

The chakra system is an energy matrix that supports physical-mental-emotional-spiritual life. *Chakra* is a Sanskrit word meaning "wheel" or disc-like spinning vortex of energy. Chakras form the coordinating network interfacing with the body through *nadis* (energy channels similar to acupuncture meridians) that directly influence the endocrine glands. Hence, they regulate and control all body functions. As we absorb more spiritual Light, energetic changes are created in our physical bodies. This energy matrix is composed of the subtle energy pathways in the body that connect the primary and secondary chakras.

The purpose of building and reinforcing an energy matrix is to handle the surges of the higher vibrational energies that are streaming forth on the planet. This energy that I am referring to is known as *prana* or *chi* in the Eastern cultures and *life force* in the Western cultures. This is the same energy that we take into our physical bodies through every breath, through raw and live foods, and walking barefoot on the land. Since the breath is by far the most common way to acquire the life-force energy, the following practices will be helpful for you to build and strengthen your energy reserves.

Of the four lower bodies, the etheric body is more aligned with the daily functioning and health of the physical body. The programming of what the physical body needs, when and where, is all built into the etheric body. It is the mysterious life force behind growth, development, and self-repairs.

Each chakra should be like a wheel moving rapidly in a clockwise rotation, and the more rapid the vibratory actions of these chakra centers in your four lower bodies, the less negativity can be absorbed through them. Since the rapid vibrations quicken the energies of the four lower bodies, depression, doubt, fear, and lethargy are more easily repelled. These negative vibrations may materialize from within your accumulations of negativity, which are recorded in your etheric body. Negative energies may also appear because they float in the atmosphere in which you move. Lastly, negative vibrations may appear because they may be consciously directed at you by others.

The chakras resemble suns of the colors of the Seven Rays, and they radiate into the individual the qualities of the Seven Rays. An overview of these Rays can be found in Chapter 14.[1] The chakras should be experienced on the physical and etheric level as wheels of Light and color, spinning outwards. They are smaller on the bottom and grow larger as they proceed up the spine, until the top chakra forms a golden yellow aura around the head.

Color Therapy

Colors can be used to assist us in concentrating and transmitting healing energies because each color is a special rate of vibration, which is its quality.[2]

Each chakra has a specific color associated with it, in the progression of the rainbow. The first chakra is red, the second is orange, the third is yellow, the fourth is green, the fifth is blue, the sixth is indigo, and the seventh is violet. An easy way to remind you of the correct colors to breathe is to purchase small colored squares of cloth of the chakra colors from a fabric store. As you lie comfortably, place the appropriately colored swatches on your chakra areas. Then as you breathe the colors into each chakra, visualize the colors being absorbed into your body to heal and to restore balance. Since all energy follows thought, the energy from the air you are breathing will automatically circulate in the way that your thoughts direct. The following technique can strengthen the vitality of each of your chakras:

- Beginning with the first chakra, breathe in the color red, through your intention or visualization. Red is stimulating, energizing, and filled with vitality and warmth. Take in as much as you need. Then hold the breath for the count of ten before you exhale. Continue breathing red into the first chakra in this manner for three or four breaths. Then go to the next chakra.

- At the second chakra, breathe in the color orange, through your intention or visualization. Orange stimulates energies, relieves depression, is joyful, and promotes well-being. Take in as much as you need. Then hold the breath for the count of ten before you exhale. Continue breathing orange into the second chakra in this manner for three or four breaths. Then go to the next chakra.

- At the third chakra, breathe in the color yellow, through your intention or visualization. Yellow stimulates the brain, is energetic, and promotes happiness. Take in as much as you need. Then hold the breath for the count of ten before you exhale. Continue breathing yellow into the third chakra in this manner for three or four breaths. Then go to the next chakra.

- At the fourth chakra, breathe in the color green, through your intention or visualization. Green is healing, peaceful, and balancing. Take in as much as you need. Then hold the breath for the count of ten before you exhale. Continue breathing green into the fourth chakra in this manner for three or four breaths. Then go to the next chakra.

- At the fifth chakra, breathe in the color blue, through your intention or visualization. Blue is calming, cooling, and relaxing. Take in as much as you need. Then hold the breath for the count of ten before you exhale. Continue breathing blue into the fifth chakra in this manner for three or four breaths. Then go to the next chakra.

- At the sixth chakra, breathe in the color indigo, through your intention or visualization. Indigo is a purifier. It sharpens intuition and is spiritual and soothing. Take in as much as you need. Then hold the breath for the count of ten before you exhale. Continue breathing indigo into the sixth chakra in this manner for three or four breaths. Then go to the next chakra.

- At the seventh chakra, breathe in the color violet, through your intention or visualization. Violet stimulates imagination and is soothing and tranquilizing. Take in as much as you need. Then hold the breath for the count of ten before you exhale. Continue breathing violet into the seventh chakra in this manner for three or four breaths.

- When finished breathing through all chakras, surround yourself with a blue bubble of Divine power that is surrounded by a gold bubble of Divine wisdom that is then surrounded by a pink bubble of Divine love. In this manner you can revitalize your body, mind, and spirit.

Chakra Breathing and Activation

In chakra breathing, you consciously direct your breath into a specific chakra. For example, first try breathing into your solar plexus chakra. As you breathe into that particular area of the body, carefully sense the motion that takes place. Feel the body gently expanding on the inhalation and contracting on the exhalation. When you have sensed the expansion and contraction clearly, you are breathing into the center. For the following exercise, you may now sense the crown and third-eye chakras in the same manner. If you are unable to sense each chakra, don't become discouraged. The ability will come with practice. In the meantime, intention is the key to directing the breath (prana) and to developing this sensitivity.

Opening the Heart Chakra

Imagine a brilliant White Light in front of you, and breathe this Light through your heart to your third eye. On the out-breath, breathe out the third eye. Continue breathing in this circular manner for a few minutes while focusing your intention on clearing away any blockages in your heart chakra.

Opening the Crown Chakra and Third Eye

Imagine the most brilliant Light conceivable, and breathe this Light in through your crown chakra and down into your pineal gland (in the very center of your head). On the out-breath, breathe the Light out through your third eye. Do this exercise for a few minutes each day to expand both the sixth and seventh chakras.

Activating Chakras

This is a powerful technique to raise your vibrations. The chakras are important doorways for the energies of each of the Seven Rays to flow. Begin this exercise by focusing your intention to breathe through each of your chakras to activate them individually. Imagine a brilliant White Light in front of you. Begin breathing this radiant Light into each chakra, starting with the root chakra and continuing up through each succeeding chakra. As you inhale, imagine the chakra being activated and opening. As you exhale the White Light, imagine that your aura is being strengthened and fortified.

As stated previously, there is a connection between the chakras and the body's endocrine gland system, and it is possible to stimulate the ductless glands through the practice of various yogic postures, through meditation, and through the use of certain seed sounds or *bijas*.[3] These bija seed sounds can be intoned as part of a process that cleanses, balances, and aligns the seven chakras prior to chanting mantras or silent meditation.[4]

- First Chakra (Muladhara, root, red color) RING LAM OM
- Second Chakra (Swadhisthana, coccyx, orange color) VANG VUM

215

- Third Chakra (Manipura, navel, yellow color) RANG RUM
- Fourth Chakra (Anahata, heart, green color) SUNG YUM
- Fifth Chakra (Vishuddi, throat, blue color) LAM OM
- Sixth Chakra (Ajna, forehead, indigo color) MUNG AUM
- Seventh Chakra (Sahasrara, crown, violet color) AUNG

Sun Meditation

This meditation can be helpful for healing the physical body, activating the spiritual bodies, and increasing your soul power. The original source of this is unknown. It can be used to heal yourself or others. In order to heal another (after you obtain their permission), picture them in the middle of the sun before you place the sun into the seventh chakra.

Sit upright in a comfortable position with your spine straight yet relaxed. Close your eyes. Relax your body. Relax the muscles behind your eyes as well. Take a deep breath and allow all of your tensions or pent-up feelings to escape. Allow yourself to become loose and relaxed.

Imagine a point between your eyebrows, inside your forehead. Now focus all your attention at this point. In your imagination, recall a scene from one of your favorite beaches as you are walking into the ocean five minutes before sunrise. As the sun rises, picture a stream of Light from the sun beaming straight to you. Now walk toward the sun on this beam of Light.

For a moment, stop and notice yourself in the middle of the ocean, standing on this beam of Light. There is only you, the sky, the water, and nothing else. Visualize your etheric soul leaving your body as it walks toward the sun and then disappears directly into it. Imagine your etheric soul sitting in a comfortable position in the middle of the sun.

Then, while looking at the sun as a large ball, imagine lifting it gently over your forehead. In your mind's eye, look at yourself looking at the sun and lifting the sun over your head with gentleness and ease.

In your imagination, notice your crown chakra (seventh chakra) opening and the sun setting within you as the crown chakra closes again. Now the center of the sun is at the level of your third eye (sixth chakra).

Pause for a few moments. Notice the total darkness and realize that you and the eternal Light of Source are merged into one.

The only thing separating you from the darkness is your body, which is a ball of fire. Now, stop a moment and notice three things:

- The darkness around you.
- You and the Light merging into one.
- Your etheric soul, sitting in the middle of the sun.

Then picture yourself as if you are looking through the opposite end of a telescope. The sun is now the size of a golf ball. The center of the sun has moved to the back of your head, touching your spinal cord. Imagine the sun now slowly moving downward until it rests at your throat chakra (fifth chakra). Watch it cleansing your throat. Feel the warmth and healing energy opening your throat chakra like a flower bud opening into a blossom. Feel the sun linger there for a few moments longer.

Then observe the sun traveling to your heart chakra (fourth chakra) and cleansing it. Feel the warmth and healing taking place in your heart, and imagine your heart center opening like the petals of a rose. Notice the warmth in your heart for a few more moments.

Staying on your spinal cord, watch the sun move above and opposite your navel,opening your solar plexus (third chakra). Feel the sun cleansing your solar plexus and the warmth, healing, and expansion of this area. Watch as the sun moves between your navel and pubic area to your sacral chakra (second chakra). Feel the opening, warmth, and cleansing of this area as well. Pause briefly as you notice the healing sensations.

Now the sun has settled at the tip of your tailbone. Stop for a while to experience the warmth, cleansing, and healing taking place in your root chakra (first chakra). Feel the entire center of the sun in this area with all its warmth. The White Light of the sun is brilliant like millions of sparkling stars. At the same time, be aware of the total darkness surrounding you like in the yin and yang symbol.

Take several deep breaths and center yourself in this root chakra area. Now watch as the sun returns to the top from the middle of your body instead of from your spine. Slowly allow it to rise and acknowledge each chakra as it returns to your third eye. At this time, picture the darkness all around you once again.

Then imagine your crown chakra opening briefly as the sun emerges. You are aglow like a multitude of fireflies in total darkness. Return the sun back to the horizon with the power of your imagination. Notice that the darkness has disappeared. Next, picture your etheric soul leaving the sun and gently returning to your body that is still standing on the ocean. As your soul merges back into your physical body, turn around and walk back to the beach. Once you've returned to the beach, turn around and glimpse the sun once again.

Fold your hands in gratitude for the healing you just received and bow your head in appreciation. Quietly state: *"Dear Source, I continue on my journey to serve humanity."* As you raise your head you will notice coming toward you a tiny white flame as a gift from Source. It now enters your third eye. Imagine that white flame glowing within your third eye. Gently open your eyes and wherever you are looking, you are looking through the white flame of Source.

Now notice if you can feel your heart beating. Be aware of the rhythm of your breath as you slowly inhale and exhale. Soon a peaceful feeling of being centered in your heart will prevail. Your heart and mind will blend as one and melt into a deeper center. It is here that you will be able to receive renewed energy and awareness.

Dr. MacDonald-Bayne's Breathing Exercise

Dr. Murdo MacDonald-Bayne, fondly referred to as Dr. Mac by his students, was a renowned spiritual teacher, author, healer, and psychic who made his transition in 1955.

The following exercise is found in his book *Spiritual and Mental Healing*. It is a very powerful method of using the breath for strengthening your energy matrix in order to carry additional life-force energy throughout your physical body. There are different rhythms in his breathing exercises. The healing breath rhythm is 8-4-8-4.

Using this 8-4-8-4 healing rhythm, inhale a breath taking eight heartbeats, hold for four heartbeats, exhale over eight heartbeats, pause for four heartbeats, and so on. You can monitor your heartbeats by placing your finger on your pulse until you can automatically judge the time. If you are unable to do the 8-4-8-4, then start with 4-2-4-2 and increase to 6-3-6-3, until you are able to acquire the 8-4-8-4 rhythm easily.

It is best to practice about ten minutes, twice daily. For best results, keep your mouth closed and breathe through your nose. However, do not strain your breathing and don't worry if you are unable to accomplish the longer breath for a while. The main thing to establish is rhythmic breathing in order to tune into the rhythm of the Universe and thereby be vitalized by the Divine Force.

When using the 8-4-8-4 rhythm, say at the same time, *"Divine Life fills me."* Feel as though you are breathing through every portion of your body to begin with; this brings the whole body in tune with the Universal Healing Power.[5]

Example:

Divine Life fills me

Inhale	1	2	3	4	5	6	7	8

Divine Life fills me

Hold	1	2	3	4

Divine Life fills me

Exhale	1	2	3	4	5	6	7	8

Divine Life fills me

Pause	1	2	3	4

Imagine that your spirit (not your body) is breathing in life-force energy as you inhale. When you exhale, imagine this energy being diffused throughout your entire physical body.

After you master the basic breathing exercise above, you can focus your attention on developing your individual energy matrix. This can be accomplished by concentrating as if you were breathing through each of the following centers:

1. The whole being at the same time while saying, "Divine Life fills me."
2. The base of the spine while saying, "Divine Vitality fills me."
3. The small of the back while saying, "Divine Strength fills me."
4. The middle of the back while saying, "Divine Power fills me."
5. Between the shoulders while saying, "Divine Love fills me."
6. Base of head while saying, "Divine Life fills me."
7. Top of head while saying, "Divine Inspiration fills me."
8. Forehead, between the eyes, while saying, "Divine Light fills me."
9. The heart while saying, "Divine Truth fills me."
10. The whole being again, this time saying, "Divine Healing fills me."

Now meditate on your Oneness with Source for thirty minutes, opening yourself to the inflow of Divine Energy. It is recommended that you practice this exercise both morning and night.

Here are more detailed instructions for the breathing exercise above:

- Begin by lying down in a comfortable position stretched out on your back. Relax yourself completely and breathe naturally for a few minutes in order to align with the Universe.

- In this exercise, breathe in for eight counts, hold your breath for four counts, exhale for eight counts, and then hold your breath for four counts. Breathe for approximately three to five minutes into each of the following energy centers.

- Start by breathing into the entire body while you simultaneously say: *"Divine Life fills me."*

- Breathe into the base of the spine at the root chakra and say: *"Divine Vitality fills me."* (As you breathe, imagine the Universal Power coursing up and down your spine.)

- Breathe into the small of the back, opposite the navel, and say: *"Divine Strength fills me."*
- Breathe into the middle of the back, opposite the solar plexus area, and say: *"Divine Power fills me."*
- Breathe into the area between the shoulders, behind the heart, and say: *"Divine Love fills me."*
- Breathe into the back of the head, at the base of the skull, and say: *"Divine Life fills me."*
- Breathe into the crown chakra, at the top of the head, and say: *"Divine Inspiration fills me."*
- Breathe into the third-eye area, between the eyebrows, and say: *"Divine Light fills me."*
- Breathe into the heart and say: *"Divine Truth fills me."*
- Breathe into the entire body again and say: *"Divine Healing fills me."*

After breathing through the entire body, sit quietly and simply meditate for thirty minutes on your oneness with Source. You can say the mantra *"I AM One with Source"* as you meditate. During this phase, do not try to force anything; simply allow yourself to relax.[6]

After traveling all over the world and studying with the finest living Masters, Dr. MacDonald-Bayne concluded that this particular exercise was one of the most powerful and transformational he had ever practiced.

Chapter 14

Awakening Your Divine Blueprint

Each of us has within a unique Divine Blueprint. It holds our life's purpose and role at this time, as well as in the Divine Plan that is the pre-laid destiny of all humanity. Destiny is discovering your unique place in this Greater Plan. Accessing this information and finding one's role is only accomplished through the inner journey of self-knowledge. All that we experience in this lifetime is part of our training and preparation for this role.[1]

As we expand our consciousness through the desire in our heart to realize our true potential, we can become more aware of the significance of our life in this incarnation. The following prayer can assist us in aligning with our Divine Blueprint.

Dear Source, I ask that the next perfect step of my piece in the Divine Plan clearly be revealed to me and bring with it the perfect people required to make this piece manifest into physical reality NOW![2]

When we access our Divine Blueprint, discover our life purpose, and fulfill that purpose, we realize that ascension is the act of tuning the vibrational frequencies of our four-body system to resonate in complete harmony with the I AM Presence within us.[3] Everything is composed of energy on this planet, and there is a synergy among our physical, emotional, mental, and spiritual bodies. Science has proven that the physical body, which seems solid, is actually composed of groups of electrons. Around those electrons, negative environmental energies can be drawn into the cellular atmosphere. Instead of having the rainbow colors as your aura, you instead might have a "clogging" of the little force fields, which has closed in the light of the electrons. Because this accumulation has been magnetized into the physical body, it has "bogged down" the vibratory action of the atoms and they no longer vibrate in harmony with your keynote. They have lost the resiliency and buoyancy that they have when they vibrate with their natural True Self.

The same thing is true of your mental body. The electrons that comprise the mental body are absorbing negative substances constantly from the atmosphere. Therefore, what your mind dwells upon secretly, you are drawing into the force fields of the electrons and atoms of your mental body and your physical form, as well as producing manifestations that may be viewed by a psychic. The vibratory action of your emotional body, if flooded with disharmony of any kind, will manifest as imperfection in the substance you have drawn into the force fields of the electrons forming the atoms that compose the emotional body. This density that is drawn in slows down their vibratory action, and consequently, emotional upheavals can occur.[4]

Divine Breathing Exercise

This breathing technique allows you to develop the feeling of Unity Consciousness. Over time, and with consistency, your consciousness will merge with All That Is. This may be done anywhere; however, prior to sleep is an excellent time. The affirmation for this exercise is *"I AM filled with the Power and Healing of God, or Source."*

- Starting with the inhalation (in-breath), repeat the affirmation to yourself two times.
- Then hold your breath (pause) for four counts and repeat the affirmation once.
- Upon exhalation (out-breath) repeat the affirmation to yourself two times.
- Then hold your breath (pause) for four counts and repeat the affirmation once.

- Meditate with the following mantra for thirty minutes: *"I AM One with God, or Source."*
- Feel your divine essence flood your mental body with the Oneness of God, or Source, as you say the mantra.
- Then move to the physical body and immerse it with the Oneness of God, or Source, as you state the mantra.
- Lastly, fill the etheric body with the Oneness of God, or Source, as you repeat the mantra.
- You may substitute the following affirmation if you desire more guidance in your life: *"I AM filled with the Power and Guidance of God, or Source."*
- For a more powerful experience, you may wish to utilize the following three-item affirmation with the breathing sequence above and state: *"I AM filled with the Power and the Guidance and the Healing of God, or Source."*[5]

Subtle Bodies

The aura is composed of four energy fields. These are the physical health aura, the emotional aura, the mental aura, and the etheric body aura. This aura radiates from all bodies in every direction. You live, move, and look out into the world through this fourfold aura.[6]

All of us have these four distinct and separate energy bodies, which interpenetrate each other and have their different unique perspectives. The physical body is located in the center and is the densest of the four lower bodies. Next to the physical body is the etheric body. Then follow the mental and emotional bodies. The subtle bodies consist of the etheric body, the mental body, and the emotional body. All these bodies have the shape of ovoids and they surround and interpenetrate your physical body. They also interpenetrate each other.

The emotional body is the largest of the four lower bodies and the subtle energy body through which feelings are created, expressed, and stored. The ego resides here. The ideal is to respect and tune into all four bodies simultaneously for insights. Unfortunately, we often tend to over-identify with one or two of the energy bodies to the detriment of the others. More than half of the people on Earth respond to life through the focus of their emotional body.[7]

Cleansing Your Four Lower Bodies

The following instruction is a daily exercise recommended by Master St. Germain. He suggests that before retiring at night you stand in your room and give the following decree:

I call forth my I AM Presence and Ascended Master St. Germain to blaze the Violet Fire into action, through and around me, in a circle nine feet in diameter.

Then raise your hands up to your I AM Presence and state:

I AM Presence and Ascended Master St. Germain, qualify these hands with the purifying power of the Violet Flame.

Do this three times.

Now, starting at your head, move your hands from above your body to your feet, passing over as much of your body surface as you can reach with your hands. (You don't actually touch the physical body.) Then with the left hand, sweep down over your right shoulder, arm, and hand. Next, with the right hand, give the left shoulder, arm, and hand the same treatment. Then shake your hands from the wrist as if you were flicking a negative substance into the surrounding Violet Fire. Do this seven times.

Master St. Germain has stated that if you could see with the inner sight what takes place in the first part of the exercise, it is though a tight-fitting garment of black substance were being removed from the body with the hands. The second time you go over the body, the garment removed is of a dark gray substance; the third time it is of a lighter gray color and so on. Night after night, as you proceed with this exercise, this astral substance gets lighter and lighter in color and texture. Finally it is removed entirely from the body and purification takes place.[8]

The Violet Fire makes each one of your four lower bodies lighter. As you consciously invoke the Violet Fire to sweep through your physical body, then your etheric, mental, and emotional bodies, it purifies the energy that may be slowing down the vibration of these bodies. The removal of this discordant energy allows the electrons in your four lower bodies to spin more rapidly, and thus they increase in vibration to be more sensitive to your I AM Presence.[9]

Harmonizing Lower Bodies

The following exercise is an adaptation of one of my Land Clearing processes. Before beginning this process, make yourself comfortable. Next take three slow deep breaths as you set your intention to remove any energy blockages that are held in your four lower bodies (physical, etheric, emotional, and mental). Then summon the Masters of the Seven Rays as follows:

I call forth the Masters and Angels of the Seven Rays to totally surround my physical, etheric, emotional, and mental bodies.

Physical Body

- Ask the Master and Angels of the Blue Ray to place a blanket of blue Light beneath your physical body and lift the blanket of blue Light straight up through your entire physical body.
- Ask that the blue blanket of Light gather up all negative energies from your physical body and take them to the Light of Source for transmutation.
- Request that the Divine Blueprint of your physical body now be restored.

Etheric Body

- Ask the Master and Angels of the Green Ray to place a blanket of green Light beneath your etheric body and lift the blanket of green Light straight up through your entire etheric body.

- Ask that the green blanket of Light gather up all negative energies from your etheric body and take them to the Light of Source for transmutation.
- Request that the Divine Blueprint of this etheric body now be restored.

Emotional Body

- Now ask the Master and Angels of the Pink Ray to place a blanket of pink Light beneath your emotional body and lift the blanket of pink Light straight up through your entire emotional body.
- Ask that the pink blanket of Light gather up all negative energies from your emotional body and take them to the Light of Source for transmutation.
- Request that the Divine Blueprint of this emotional body now be restored.

Mental Body

- Ask the Master and Angels of the Gold Ray to place a blanket of gold Light beneath your mental body and lift the blanket of gold Light straight up through your entire mental body.
- Ask that the gold blanket of Light gather up all negative energies from your mental body and take them to the Light of Source for transmutation.
- Request that the Divine Blueprint of this mental body now be restored.

The last step of this process is to request that any and all voids created by the release of all these discordant energies be filled with White Light and Unconditional Love. Then thank the Masters and Angels of the Seven Rays for all the healing that you received.

The Three-Fold Flame

The Three-Fold Flame is the perfect integration of love (pink), wisdom (gold), and power (blue) that resides in the heart center and creates comfort, healing, peace, truth, and transmutation. Within that tiny Flame is the power to generate the energy to disintegrate any amount of discordant energy. The action is similar to that of a wire transmitting electricity to light an entire building or a city.[10]

One action of the Three-Fold Flame that can be implemented is to draw any negativity of each of the subtle bodies into the Flame in the heart and command that it be consumed. You can also imagine and feel a large Three-Fold Flame around the physical body that resembles three ostrich plumes or stalks of pampas grass, extending from beneath your feet to a foot or so above your head, with the blue plume at the left side, slightly to the back, the gold one in front, and the pink one at the right, meeting the blue one at the center back.[11]

Call forth your I AM Presence to balance the Three-Fold Flame in your heart.

1. Begin this exercise by reestablishing a slow, rhythmic breath.

2. Place your physical body in a relaxed but poised position with your back straight, yet carrying no tension in any muscles.

3. As the rhythmic breath continues, begin to relax into the intensity of Light coming from within your heart.

4. See or imagine an ever-expanding, spiraling, upward-rushing combined Flame of Love, Wisdom, and Power. The Three-Fold Flame is the energy of Divine power, Divine wisdom, and Divine love. Its three plumes are blue, gold, and pink and it resides in your heart. Visualize or feel it spiraling up from your physical heart center, increasing the entire vibratory action of the physical body structure with expansion.

5. Next, focus your attention on the etheric heart center and notice again the Three-Fold Flame expanding through your entire etheric body.

6. See the heart of your mental body with the Three-Fold Flame expanding there and accelerating the substance of the brain matter, etheric mind, and mental body into shimmering Light substance that carries the perfect ideas of Source ... crystal-line clear. Pause for a moment to experience it all.

7. Now include the great heart center of your emotional body, feeling the Three-Fold Flame expanding through every cell,

molecule, and atom of the great sea of your emotional world.

8. Then visualize each of the Three-Fold Flames blending as one gigantic spiraling Three-Fold Flame, an upward rushing force of vibration and consciousness unifying each of the four lower bodies. Visualize them all in the perfect pattern of your Divine Blueprint: not as shapeless ovoids of Light but as glowing Beings of Light, one aligned with the other ... all in perfect harmony ... in perfect Unity.

9. Now feel each breath expanding to the depth of each of your four lower bodies, for it is the same Source energy that is emanating from each one ... all now under the control of the I AM Presence. Follow with a silent period.[12]

Three-Fold Flame Breathing

Once you have visualized the Three-Fold Flame, the *next step is to seal yourself and your consciousness in a globe of White Fire*. This is another powerful exercise to strengthen your energy circuits and increase your vibratory rate. It would be most helpful if you set these goals as your intention before you begin each practice.

- Find a comfortable place to sit or lie down, where you will be undisturbed.
- Call forth Archangel Michael, who represents Divine Power, three times.
- Call forth Archangel Jophiel, who represents Divine Wisdom, three times.
- Call forth Archangel Chamuel, who represents Divine Love, three times.
- Now imagine that Archangel Michael (Blue Ray) is standing to your left.
- Imagine that Archangel Jophiel (Gold Ray) is standing directly in front.
- Imagine that Archangel Chamuel (Pink Ray) is standing to your right.
- Visualize Blue Light streaming toward you from Archangel Michael.

- Visualize Gold Light streaming toward you from Archangel Jophiel.
- Visualize Pink Light streaming toward you from Archangel Chamuel.
- Next, with focus and intention, breathe this powerful color combination, known as the Three-Fold Flame, into your chakras.
- Inhale the Three-Fold Flame of colors into the front of your root chakra.
- Pause briefly, and then exhale the colors out the back of your root chakra.
- Hold your breath now to the count of four, imagining the chakra opening.
- Continue this rhythm of breathing the Three-Fold Flame into the front of each chakra, pausing, and then exhaling the color out the back of each chakra.
- Repeat this breathing sequence for your navel, solar plexus, heart, throat, third eye, and crown chakras.
- After breathing through each individual chakra, imagine a brilliant, shimmering Green Light flowing up from the Earth into your root chakra.
- This brilliant Green Light continues flowing up through your spine to your crown chakra and then cascades down the front of your body.
- Continue breathing this shimmering Green Light up through your chakras and spine, over your crown, and down the front of your body for four complete cycles.
- Try to breathe the Green Light completely from the root to the crown with one uninterrupted breath.
- After you complete the exercise, you can revisit any chakras where you want to provide more concentration.

It will be your focus, intuition, and practice that will make this exercise the most successful.

Infusion of Seven Rays

A Ray in this context is a type of energy containing a specific quality or attribute. The Ray forces are believed to enter our solar system by emanation from the Great Central Sun, a larger metaphysical sun that exists beyond our solar system. It is the sun behind our sun in the center of our galaxy. From this Central Sun, the energies radiate to the core of the Earth. From the center of the Earth's core, Ray forces radiate to the Earth's surface. Each Ascended Master is identified with a Ray force when in service as a Master Teacher to humanity. The qualities and attributes of their teachings reflect the energies of that particular Ray. For human beings on their spiritual path, the use of the Rays brings healing to many aspects of life: relationships, career, money, and health.[13]

Each of the Seven Rays embodies a certain type of energy. An individual can call forth whatever type of energy is required at any given time. For instance, if you desire more will power, you can call forth the First Ray; if you want more wisdom, you can call forth the Second Ray; if you want more devotion, you can summon the Sixth Ray. If you want to evoke the Violet Fire, you can call forth the Seventh Ray. Depending on which quality you desire, all you need to do is say (silently or verbally): "I now call forth the _____ Ray." A Ray can be requested by the number, color, quality, or energy. The particular energy will flow in instantly, no matter where you are in your spiritual evolution. All you need to do is request it.[14]

The Seven Basic Rays, and the chakras they affect, are as follows:

1. **Blue Ray:** Throat Chakra
2. **Gold Ray:** Crown
3. **Pink Ray:** Heart Chakra
4. **White Ray:** Base of the Spine
5. **Green Ray:** Third Eye
6. **Gold Ruby Ray:** Solar Plexus Chakra
7. **Violet Ray:** Seat of the Soul

The Ascended Masters included in this practice are each responsible for a specific Ray and thereby possess all the qualities of that particular Ray. Full possession of the qualities of one Ray does not imply a lack of the qualities of the other Rays.[15]

Following are brief introductions to each of these Ascended Masters of the Seven Rays.

Master El Morya
He is the representative of the First Ray of Strength.

Master Kuthumi
He was formerly the great teacher Pythagoras and now represents the Second Ray, which is the Ray of Wisdom.

Paul the Venetian
He is at the Head of the Third Ray. The characteristic of Adaptability is strongly associated with this Master.

Master Serapis Bey
The Fourth Ray is under his care and introduces Harmony and Art into the environment.

Master Hilarion
At the Head of the Fifth Ray, he represents Science (scientific accuracy).

Lady Master Nada
She is a member of the Karmic Board and rules the Sixth Ray of Devotion.

Master St. Germain
He is the Master of the Seventh Ray of Service. In a recent lifetime he was previously known as Sir Francis Bacon.[16]

Begin by calling forth the Ascended Masters of the Seven Rays: Master El Morya, Master Kuthumi, Paul the Venetian, Master Serapis Bey, Master Hilarion, Lady Master Nada, and Master St. Germain.

Imagine that all the Masters are surrounding you in a circle. Visualize, feel, or imagine the energy of each Ray flowing through your entire body, beginning with your physical body. Through your intention, imagine that energy flows through your chakras (both front and back) to flood your entire etheric body. Then request that the energy flow through your chakras to your emotional body, fully immersing it. Finally request that the energy flow through your chakras to totally fill up your mental body. At this time, your auric field will become a bright ball of energy that is evenly distributed throughout your physical, etheric, emotional, and mental bodies.

The First Ray: Power, Faith, Protection

I now call forth the Master of the Blue Ray, Master El Morya, and ask that my physical body be infused with the vibrations and divine qualities of the color Blue. (Imagine your physical body being flooded with the powerful energy of the color blue.)

I now request that the energy and vitality of the Blue Ray flow through each of my chakras and then into my etheric body. (Visualize the energy flooding through the front and back of all your chakras, including those in your hands and feet, then filling up your etheric body.)

I now request that the energy and vitality of the Blue Ray flow through each of my chakras and then into my emotional body. (Visualize the energy flooding through the front and back of all your chakras, including those in your hands and feet, then filling up your emotional body.)

I now request that the energy and vitality of the Blue Ray flow through each of my chakras and then into my mental body. (Visualize the energy flooding through the front and back of all your chakras, including those in your hands and feet, then filling up your mental body.)

For a moment, notice the sensation of the Blue Ray flowing through and revitalizing your physical body, all your chakras, your etheric body, your emotional body, and your mental body. Just visualize or imagine that this energy is circulating throughout your entire energy system.[17]

The Second Ray: Wisdom, Illumination, Perception

I now call forth the Master of the Gold Ray, Master Kuthumi, and ask that my physical body be infused with the vibrations and divine qualities of the color Gold. (Imagine your physical body being flooded with the powerful energy of the Gold Ray.)

I now request that the energy and vitality of the Gold Ray flow through each of my chakras and then into my etheric body. (Visualize the energy flooding through the front and back of all your chakras, including those in your hands and feet, then filling up your etheric body.)

I now request that the energy and vitality of the Gold Ray flow through each of my chakras and then into my emotional body. (Visualize the energy flooding through the front and back of all your chakras, including those in your hands and feet, then filling up your emotional body.)

I now request that the energy and vitality of the Gold Ray flow through each of my chakras and then into my mental body. (Visualize the energy flooding through the front and back of all your chakras, including those in your hands and feet, then filling up your mental body.)[18]

The Third Ray: Divine Love, Compassion, Forgiveness

I now call forth the Master of the Pink Ray, Paul the Venetian, and ask that my physical body be infused with the vibrations and divine qualities of the color Pink. (Imagine your physical body being flooded with the powerful energy of the Pink Ray.)

I now request that the energy and vitality of the Pink Ray flow through each of my chakras and then into my etheric body. (Visualize the energy flooding through the front and back of all your chakras, including those in your hands and feet, then filling up your etheric body.)

I now request that the energy and vitality of the Pink Ray flow through each of my chakras and then into my emotional body. (Visualize the energy flooding through the front and back of all your chakras, including those in your hands and feet, then filling up your emotional body.)

I now request that the energy and vitality of the Pink Ray flow through each of my chakras and then into my mental body. (Visualize the energy flooding through the front and back of all your chakras, including those in your hands and feet, then filling up your mental body.)[19]

The Fourth Ray: Purity, Wholeness, Ascension

I now call forth the Master of the White Ray, Master Serapis Bey, and ask that my physical body be infused with the vibrations and divine qualities of the color White. (Imagine your physical body being flooded with the powerful energy of the White Ray.)

I now request that the energy and vitality of the White Ray flow through each of my chakras and then into my etheric body. (Visualize the energy flooding through the front and back of all your chakras, including those in your hands and feet, then filling up your etheric body.)

I now request that the energy and vitality of the White Ray flow through each of my chakras and then into my emotional body. (Visualize the energy flooding through the front and back of all your chakras, including those in your hands and feet, then filling up your emotional body.)

I now request that the energy and vitality of the White Ray flow through each of my chakras and then into my mental body. (Visualize the energy flooding through the front and back of all your chakras, including those in your hands and feet, then filling up your mental body.)[20]

The Fifth Ray: Healing, Manifestation, Truth

I now call forth the Master of the Green Ray, Master Hilarion, and ask that my physical body be infused with the vibrations and divine qualities of the color Green. (Imagine your physical body being flooded with the powerful energy of the Green Ray.)

I now request that the energy and vitality of the Green Ray flow through each of my chakras and then into my etheric body. (Visualize the energy flooding through the front and back of all your chakras, including those in your hands and feet, then filling up your etheric body.)

I now request that the energy and vitality of the Green Ray flow through each of my chakras and then into my emotional body. (Visualize the energy flooding through the front and back of all your chakras, including those in your hands and feet, then filling up your emotional body.)

I now request that the energy and vitality of the Green Ray flow through each of my chakras and then into my mental body. (Visualize the energy flooding through the front and back of all your chakras, including those in your hands and feet, then filling up your mental body.)[21]

The Sixth Ray: Devotion, Service, Peace

I now call forth the Master of the Gold Ruby Ray, Lady Master Nada, and ask that my physical body be infused with the vibrations and divine qualities of the color Gold Ruby. (Imagine your physical body being flooded with the powerful energy of the Gold Ruby Ray.)

I now request that the energy and vitality of the Gold Ruby Ray flow through each of my chakras and then into my etheric body. (Visualize the energy flooding through the front and back of all your chakras, including those in your hands and feet, then filling up your etheric body.)

I now request that the energy and vitality of the Gold Ruby Ray flow through each of my chakras and then into my emotional body. (Visualize the energy flooding through the front and back of all your chakras, including those in your hands and feet, then filling up your emotional body.)

I now request that the energy and vitality of the Gold Ruby Ray flow through each of my chakras and then into my mental body. (Visualize the energy flooding through the front and back of all your chakras, including those in your hands and feet, then filling up your mental body.)[22]

The Seventh Ray: Transmutation, Freedom, Transformation

I now call forth the Master of the Violet Ray, Master St. Germain, and ask that my physical body be infused with the vibrations and divine qualities of the color Violet. (Imagine your physical body being flooded with the powerful energy of the Violet Ray.)

I now request that the energy and vitality of the Violet Ray flow through each of my chakras and then into my etheric body. (Visualize the energy flooding through the front and back of all your chakras, including those in your hands and feet, then filling up your etheric body.)

I now request that the energy and vitality of the Violet Ray flow through each of my chakras and then into my emotional body. (Visualize the energy flooding through the front and back of all your chakras, including those in your hands and feet, then filling up your emotional body.)

I now request that the energy and vitality of the Violet Ray flow through each of my chakras and then into my mental body. (Visualize the energy flooding through the front and back of all your chakras, including those in your hands and feet, then filling up your mental body.)

After infusing the four lower bodies with the Seven Rays, make the following request to balance your entire being with the vibrations and to infuse your thoughts, words, and actions with the Seven Rays as follows:

I call upon all the Masters of the Seven Rays to balance my four lower bodies with Your vibrations. I request that the gifts of the Seven Rays and their divine qualities be activated within me now. Thank you.[23]

For those who want to learn more about the aspects, attributes, and use of the Seven Rays, I recommend reading Aurelia Louise Jones's book *The Seven Sacred Flames.*[24]

Chapter 15

Spiritual Growth Exercises

The following additional exercises have been included to assist you further on your spiritual path.

Heart Center Awakening

Healing and opening the heart is a key to awakening the spirit within you. This exercise will help you to develop heart consciousness, which entails releasing old values, concepts, and beliefs that keep you tethered and prevent you from establishing a connection with All That Is. The original source of this meditation is unknown.

1. Find a place where you can be comfortable and undisturbed.
2. Allow your eyes to close gently, and focus your attention on your heart center in the middle of your chest.
3. In your imagination, shrink yourself so you can enter your heart. Upon entering, notice that before you is a temple on the top of a hill. This is the Temple of the Heart.
4. Climb the steps to the top of the hill and enter the center doorway. Once inside, notice the appearance of this temple. Is it well kept and cleaned? Or is it full of dust and cobwebs?
5. Walk into the dimly lit interior and move to the central altar. As you approach the light at the altar, be aware of a flickering light within you. The closer you come to the altar, the brighter the flame grows. The flames merge and become one.
6. Take a moment to gaze at this flame. Send it loving energy and observe it growing brighter in response until it reaches up

to touch the ceiling forty feet above. You are feeling the flame of your heart and stimulating it to grow.

7. Breathe in and out deeply and realize in the depths of your soul that your heart center is coming alive.

8. Pay attention to the warm and joyful countenance you are experiencing while stimulating and expanding your heart center and strengthening your connection with your Higher Self.

9. When you are ready, open your eyes and sit quietly to reflect on this feeling of balance and centeredness for five minutes before ending the session.[1]

Master St. Germain's Breathing Instructions

The following three breathing exercises were taught by Master St. Germain in the 1940s. It is believed that the use of these breaths on a regular basis will assist in increasing a person's vibrations and balancing the physical body.

Through your intention you can draw forth into your body, through your breath, any particular qualities that you place your attention on. These could include: love, joy, clarity, peace, harmony, wisdom, trust, creativity, abundance, faith, and perfect health, to name a few. With greater relaxation in your emotional body, the Light will flow into you more readily without interruption.

Give all these breaths an even count—either two, four, six, or eight, depending upon the length of time you can comfortably hold the breath; then as you progress you can increase the count. As you use these techniques, focus your attention on your I AM Presence as you issue a decree that has an even number of syllables or counts within it, such as:

I AM all Light (four counts)
I AM the Violet Fire (six counts)

Use whatever decree resonates with you as long as it has an even number of syllables. You can use longer decrees as you are able to hold the breath longer.

Balancing Breath

This particular breathing exercise is especially helpful if you are experiencing physical pain anywhere in your body.

Hold your right nostril closed and inhale a deep breath through your left nostril as you state the decree. Then hold your breath while you again state the decree. Exhale through your right nostril, stating your decree as you do so. Then hold your breath for the same length of time, stating your decree. Feel and imagine a Golden Flame flowing through every cell of your body from head to toe. As it passes through your physical body, visualize that the Golden Flame then surrounds your entire body like a Golden Sun.

Repeat this exercise through the right nostril and keep alternating until you have repeated the exercise as many times as is comfortable. You will be able to increase the counts and find a balance coming into your body that has not been there before.

Energizing Breath

Regardless of how tired you may be, you will find that this breathing exercise energizes the entire body.

Take a slow deep breath, filling the lungs; hold for a moment to issue your decree; then exhale very slowly (like you are going to whistle, but you don't). Repeat this process ten or twenty times regardless of how tired you may be. You will find that it energizes the entire body. Always do this breathing exercise while keeping your focus on your I AM Presence and stating your decrees with each inhalation and exhalation. This exercise can be done as you are walking, riding, or any other activity of your choice.

Rhythmic Breath

Anyone who does these three breaths as given will find their body feeling more balanced.

Mentally say the decree on the inhalation of air into your lungs; hold for an equal number of counts; state your decree again; exhale and state your decree; hold again for an equal length of time and state your decree. Repeat this exercise several times to begin with, until you feel a balance coming from your body. You can increase the count as you progress in holding your breath longer. However, do not hold your breath at any time longer than is comfortable.[2]

Attuning to Fifth-Dimensional Energies

Our bodies' frequencies are speeding up so that we can step into the higher fifth-dimensional frequencies. This exercise helps you adjust to these energies, using Chinese concepts of energy channels or meridians in the human body.

There are multiple energy channels in the physical body, but the most important ones are the front channel that runs vertically through the middle front of the body, known as the Conception Vessel Meridian, and the back channel that runs along the spine to the head, called the Governing Vessel Meridian. All other channels interface with these two major channels. A blockage in either of them can cause many problems in the physical body.

The following is one technique, done standing vertically, for aligning and integrating with the new—higher and more rapid—energy vibrations. I have adapted it from my practice of Spring Forest Qigong as taught by Master Chunyi Lin.[3]

1. Stand with your feet about shoulder width apart. Place your tongue against the roof of your mouth. This gesture serves as a switch that connects the two major energy channels mentioned above.

2. Relax your arms at your side and slowly take a deep breath. Slowly, inhale and exhale into your abdomen until you feel a sense of peace or calmness filling your body. This may take several minutes.

3. Now imagine that you can use your entire body to breathe. In your mind's eye, visualize radiating and shimmering Universal energy permeating every cell of your body with every inhalation.

4. As you exhale, visualize or feel any pain, illness, discomfort, or areas of tension oozing out of all the cells of your body, like black puffs of smoke returning back to the Universe to be transmuted.

5. Continue this cycle of breathing for two or three minutes.

6. Next, inhale and visualize this Universal energy replenishing every part of your body, mind, and spirit with healing and rejuvenation. Exhale completely.

7. Inhale again, filling any painful or empty areas with this energy.

8. Then close your eyes and mentally say:

I AM in the fifth-dimensional energy.
The fifth-dimensional energy is in my mind, body, and spirit.
The fifth-dimensional energy and I are merging.
The fifth-dimensional energy is integrating within me, with ease and grace, at the pace that is best for me for my highest good.

Continue this process for several minutes until you feel in harmony with your surroundings. Now gently focus on your heart center (in the middle of your chest) for a few breaths and nourish your whole Being with the vibration of love. Then slowly open your eyes, noticing the stillness within and around you.

Short Version

1. Simply feel your fifth-dimensional energy around you, like clothing.

2. Focus your intent on the fifth-dimensional energy self.

3. Breathe in the fifth-dimensional energy frequency.

4. As you breathe it in, say with each breath: *"I AM fifth-dimensional."*

5. It is recommended that you do this process for twenty minutes a day.[4]

Chapter 16

Earth Healings

These healings for Mother Earth can all be woven into a daily spiritual practice, if you desire to assist the Earth in Her ascension.

Prayer for the Removal of Fear

The original source of this prayer for all humanity is unknown. Perhaps it is a prayer you'll want to add to your daily practice.

Take three deep breaths. Center yourself and then state the following:

I call forth: My I AM Presence; the Source of All That Is; the Masters of the Seven Rays; Angels of the Violet Fire; Archangels Michael, Gabriel, Uriel, Raphael; Mother Earth; the Deva of the Earth Kingdom; Pan and the Nature Spirits; and the Elemental Beings of Fire, Air, Water, and Earth.

I ask for the continuous removal of all core fear related to lack of money and financial resources for all Beings living on the planet and the general fear of a global economic meltdown. Please replace this financial fear with abundance, prosperity, and love of Source for all humanity on Earth, if it is for the highest good of all residing on this planet.

Flood the Earth with Violet Fire

I call forth: My I AM Presence; the Source of All That Is; the Masters of the Seven Rays; Angels of the Violet Fire; Archangels Michael, Gabriel, Uriel, Raphael; Mother Earth; the Deva of the Earth Kingdom; Pan and the Nature Spirits; and the Elemental Beings of Fire, Air, Water, and Earth.

I ask that the Earth and all of evolution be saturated with limitless waves of Violet Fire. I call for all negativity and activities on Earth that are not reflecting the highest Light and the holy purposes of Source to be miraculously swept and transformed, by the power of the Violet Flame, into Divine love and harmony for the restoration of Earth and humankind to the blueprint of perfection that was originally intended. May Peace and Love be spread throughout the Earth each and every day and in every way.

I give thanks that it is done now, according to the Holy Will of Source! So be it, so be it, so be it![1]

Decrees for Mother Earth

Say each of the following decrees aloud three times.

1. *Expand, expand, expand, and intensify daily the most powerful action of the Violet Fire in, through, and around the cause and core of the source of all doubt, fear, greed, and anger in the Earth, on the Earth, and in its atmosphere.*[2]

2. *Blaze, blaze, blaze and expand, expand, expand the Violet Transmuting Flame in, through, and around the Planet Earth and all the inhabitants.*[3]

3. *Blaze, blaze, blaze and expand, expand, expand the Violet Transmuting Flame in, through, and around all our governments at the local, state, and national levels and through all governments on Earth until Eternal Peace manifests and is eternally sustained.*[4]

246

Healing Prayer for Mother Earth

I call forth the spirits of the natural world: the Devas for earth, air, fire and water; the Devas and nature spirits for trees, plants, animals, and for the oceans and skies. I call for the Violet Flame of purification and forgiveness from Master St. Germain to come from the core of the Earth and sweep with a great blazing glory through every atom of the planet, every heart and mind, all of life, everything! I affirm that all thought-forms available for healing together with all dark energies of the lower astral plane are lifted so that the lower-density vibrations may be elevated and transmuted in Divine love and light.

I send love and healing energies to all of Mother Earth. I send blessings to the waters—brooks, rivers, lakes, seas, oceans. I see them totally cleansed and pure.

Take the time to see and feel all these healings. It is especially powerful to visualize brilliant Light through each aspect.[5]

Violet Flame Infusion

I AM the Violet Flame blazing, blazing through me now.

I AM the Violet Flame infusing each one of my chakras.

I AM the Violet Flame activating each strand of my DNA.

I AM the Violet Flame erasing all human imperfection.

I AM the Violet Flame enfolding me with the Love of Mother/ Father God.

State:

Violet Flame, Violet Flame, Violet Flame, may you flood this entire planet and all of humanity in an auric field of your Light, freeing and transforming all that is less than Source's perfection! So be it, so be it, so be it![6]

Energy Clearing for Natural Disasters

The following decrees, adapted from Electrons and the Elemental Kingdom (a book about the Elemental Beings),[7] are designed to restore a harmonious relationship between humanity and the Elemental Beings inhabiting the four elements of nature: air, water, earth, and fire. These decrees are valuable tools to prevent (or at least mitigate and lessen) the effect of earthquakes, forest fires, volcanic eruptions, hurricanes, floods, and tornadoes. When you give the following decrees voluntarily directed to the higher realms, the Ascended Masters may utilize the energies and increase them to transmute the root cause of the discordant use of energy by humanity.

The Air Element

The Air Element is essential for the maintenance of life on the physical plane. Its beneficial activity is seen in warm and cool breezes to propel boats, ships, and airplanes.[8]

Decree for the Air Element

I call forth my I AM Presence, anchored in my heart, and the Masters of the Seven Rays. I thank and bless all Elemental Beings of the Air Element for their past and present services.

I call on the Law of Forgiveness for myself and all humanity for all discord and disharmonious energy inflicted upon the Air Elementals by humanity for many ages.

Archangel Michael, lock your Circle and Sword of Blue Flame in, through, and around this discord and its cause, core, record, effect, and memory. Replace it with loving trust between humanity and Air Elementals. Dissolve forever the desire and capacity of humanity to use the air for destructive purposes.

Blaze! Blaze! Blaze the most dynamic action of the Violet Transmuting Flame in the form of a large Cross from the heart of the planet up, in, through, and around the Earth, all the way through to its atmosphere for at least ten thousand feet, purifying, illuminating, and healing all life on this planet and transmuting all energies into Divine love.

Free all elemental life from aversion toward humankind, leading all elemental life to the state of perfection that Source intended for it. See to it that never again will the Air Elementals participate in tornadoes, hurricanes, or any other destructive activity. What I ask for myself, I ask for all humanity, and I fully accept the fulfillment of this decree.[9]

The Earth Element

The Earth Element is vital for the production of food to assist humanity with adequate nutrition. Its beneficial action is visible in the beautiful landscapes, in flowers, in minerals, and in the production of bountiful harvests.[10]

Decree for the Earth Element

I call forth my I AM Presence, anchored in my heart, and the Masters of the Seven Rays. I thank and bless all Elemental Beings of the Earth Element for their past and present services.

I call on the Law of Forgiveness for myself and all humanity for all discord and disharmonious energy inflicted upon the Earth Elementals by humanity for many ages.

Archangel Michael, lock your Circle and Sword of Blue Flame in, through, and around this negativity and its cause, core, record, effect, and memory. Replace it with loving trust between humanity and Earth Elementals. Dissolve forever the desire and capacity of humanity to use the Earth, including the riches of her natural resources, for destructive purposes.

Blaze! Blaze! Blaze the most dynamic action of the Violet Transmuting Flame in the form of a large Cross from the heart of the planet up, in, through, and around the Earth, all the way through to its atmosphere for at least ten thousand feet, purifying, illuminating, and healing all life on this planet and transmuting all energies into Divine love.

In your cosmic authority, control all the energy of the gas belts within the Earth and transmute, transmute, transmute it all. Replace it with golden Light substance, becoming pure metallic gold that radiates through and purifies all substance not of the Light. Transmute all discord placed by humanity upon Earth Elementals and release them back into divine service.

Free every nature spirit from all destructive influences of humanity, and from the remembrance of such association and activities.

Free all elemental life from aversion toward humanity, leading all elemental life to the state of perfection that Source intended for it. See to it that never again will the Earth Elementals participate in earthquakes or any other destructive activity. What I ask for myself, I ask for all humanity, and I fully accept the fulfillment of this decree.[11]

The Water Element

The Water Element is related to the emotional body. In the physical plane, it is a great cleansing agent and one of the factors for the balancing of the weather conditions and the production of food sources.[12]

Decree for the Water Element

I call forth my I AM Presence, anchored in my heart, and the Masters of the Seven Rays. I thank and bless all Elemental Beings of the Water Element for their past and present services.

I call on the Law of Forgiveness for myself and all humanity for all discord and disharmonious energy inflicted upon the Water Elementals by humanity for many ages.

Archangel Michael, lock your Circle and Sword of Blue Flame in, through, and around this discord and its cause, core, record, effect, and memory. Replace it with loving trust between humanity and Water Elementals. Dissolve forever the desire and capacity of humanity to use the Water Element for destructive purposes.

Blaze! Blaze! Blaze the most dynamic action of the Violet Transmuting Flame in the form of a large Cross from the heart of the planet up, in, through, and around the Earth, all the way through to its atmosphere for at least ten thousand feet, purifying, illuminating, and healing all life on this planet and transmuting all energies into Divine love.

Free all elemental life from aversion toward humanity, leading all elemental life to the state of perfection that Source intended for it. See to it that never again will the Water Elementals participate in catastrophic floods or any other destructive activity. What I ask for myself, I ask for all humanity, and I fully accept the fulfillment of this decree.[13]

The Fire Element

The Fire Element is the most important of the four, as it is an expression of the Sacred Fire, from which the Violet Flame and all other flames manifest. One of its constructive activities in the physical plane is that of purification of wastes and human bodies, which allows the elements to return to the Universe.[14]

Decree for the Fire Element

I call forth my I AM Presence, anchored in my heart, and the Masters of the Seven Rays. I thank and bless all Elemental Beings of the Fire Element for their past and present services.

I call on the Law of Forgiveness for myself and all humanity for all discord and disharmonious energy inflicted upon the Fire Elementals by humanity for many ages.

Archangel Michael, lock your Circle and Sword of Blue Flame in, through, and around this discord and its cause, core, record, effect, and memory. Remove all fear of fire and transmute it into illumination and understanding of the use of the Sacred Fire. Replace it with loving trust between humanity and Fire Elementals.

Dissolve forever the desire and capacity of humanity to use the Fire Element for destructive purposes.

Blaze! Blaze! Blaze the most dynamic action of the Violet Transmuting Flame in the form of a large Cross from the heart of the planet up, in, through, and around the Earth, all the way through to its atmosphere for at least ten thousand feet, purifying, illuminating, and healing all life on this planet and transmuting all energies into Divine love.

Free all elemental life from aversion toward humanity, leading all elemental life to the state of perfection that Source intended for it. See to it that never again will the Fire Elementals participate in forest fires or any other destructive activity. What I ask for myself, I ask for all humanity, and I fully accept the fulfillment of this decree.[15]

Earth Clearings

Imagine how much negativity is being held by most pieces of land. Violent weather is Nature's way to release and transmute humanity's negative creations that are held hostage within the land. It is time to free Nature from the burden of taking care of our emotional and psychic pollution. It is time now to free the land of the negativity it has held for us and take responsibility for the transmutation of our negativity that has been imprinted within the Earth. The Violet Transmuting Flame is an excellent tool for this transmutation process. It can cleanse the physical dimension of land, including the atmosphere over the land, of all emotional and mental negativity. Land, like individuals, has an etheric body where all the events that have ever occurred on that particular piece of land are recorded. The Violet Fire has the ability to cleanse the etheric body of land so that only the constructive memories remain recorded.

Spiritual Clearing of a Lake

Following is the process that I used to release negativity held within a lake. This same process can be adapted for other bodies of water, vacant land, mountains, and National Parks. For clearing your home or personal space, or other occupied space, see Chapter 4.

Center yourself and take three deep breaths.

Evoke the presence of each Being of Light to come forth for the healing of the specific location.

State aloud:

> *I call upon Mother/Father God [or Source], the Deva of this lake*
> *[or location], the Archangels of the Four Directions (east, west,*
> *north, south), the Deva of the entire geographical region, Mother*
> *Earth (Gaia), Pan and the Nature Spirits, the Four Elements (fire,*
> *air, earth, and water), and my Guides and Teachers of 100% pure*
> *Light.*

Next evoke the Violet Transmuting Flame in order that the Pink Ray of Divine love may blaze forth. State:

> *In the name of the Master and Angels of the Violet Ray, I decree*
> *the full momentum of the Violet Flame to blaze and whirl through*
> *this lake [or location], as well as the area of land under and sur-*
> *rounding it, and transmute all negatively qualified energy into*
> *unconditional love. I decree that the Violet Flame also blaze and*
> *surround the space above the entire area for three miles upward.*

Then release any negative residual energies. State:

> *I now decree that all entities and remaining accumulated negative*
> *energies be released, blessed, and sent to the Light now!*

That statement is to be made with great intent and passion.

Proceed by filling the voids created by the releases with the Pink Ray of Divine love. State:

> *I decree that the Pink Ray of Divine love blaze through this entire*
> *area, filling every void with unconditional love.*

Continue by invoking healing for the site. State:

> *I now call upon the Divine Beings assisting with this Spiritual*
> *Clearing to remove any additional negative imprints of humanity*
> *from this lake [location] and around this lake [location] to restore*
> *the Divine blueprint of the area to its original condition. I call*

upon Mother Earth to harmonize all these energies to maximize the healing for this area. I call upon the Devas of all the Nature Kingdoms (plant, mineral, animal) to continue and sustain the work that has taken place today.

Individually thank all the Spiritual Beings who assisted you with the geographical cleansing:

Thank you Mother/Father God [or Source], the Deva of this lake [or location], the Archangels of the Four Directions (east, west, north, south), the Deva of the entire geographical region, Mother Earth (Gaia), Pan and the Nature Spirits, the Four Elements (fire, air, earth, and water), and my Guides and Teachers of 100% pure Light for assisting me with this Spiritual Clearing.

Chapter 17

Sustaining Change

Creating change in the short term is easy. Sustaining positive changes that are enduring is the challenge. Being successful will depend on your level of commitment and determination to alter the course of your life's path. Your dedication is essential to continue your progress, even if you have only a glimpse of what you are to do. Maintain the faith when interferences occur along the way. There is always a reason, as Divine timing is at work. At these times, it is best always to find something of value from everything and to determine the lesson within the experience. Sometimes all you can do is trust the process. That will help you get where you ultimately wish to be.

Maintain the faith when doors are not opening for you as you imagined they would, knowing that it is for a reason. It may be because at some level you are or were not ready to walk through them emotionally or spiritually. At other times the Universe may need additional time to arrange a sequence of events to grant your individual requests. This is simply Divine timing in action. We often are so focused on our single little door opening that we forget that every single event in the Universe is integrally connected with every other event. Each shift of energy must be considered in the grand scheme of life that is much more far-reaching than our single door.

Choosing to pursue another direction will require a serious commitment. Being successful will depend on your unwavering focus on the goal you set and breaking the many habits that have formed around the role you are leaving behind. Embrace the changes in every phase of your life and allow your True Self to unfold more fully every day in every way.

Through your choices, actions, and thoughts, you can be successful in reducing stress and increasing your spiritual pursuits. You may have already incorporated yoga, prayer, spiritual power tools, or meditation into your daily routine. You may be successfully living one day at a time and in each present moment. Your new focus is on understanding rather than being understood, and on loving rather than being loved. You practice mindfulness, chant, and issue decrees. When you are with someone, you commit to being with that person fully. When you are working on a project, you concentrate on doing that project and forget about everything else. Stress is no longer an issue. You have changed!

It has been said many times that we grow spiritually either through pain or through awareness. Take time to review the lessons gleaned from all the changes you've endured. How have you grown because of what you experienced? Support yourself. Celebrate your victories. Offer gratitude. Continue to dream of future changes. Life is change.

Trust your guidance and act on that information. As you may know, there are doors of opportunity provided within the Universe, and it is important to be aware and to act when those doors open. Pay attention, use your intuition, and walk through the doors when it is time for you to go, and know that all is in Divine Order.

Sustaining the new higher frequency and connection to Unity Consciousness will require daily attention until you are able to hold the greater Light consistently and thereby vibrate at the increased frequency rate to activate your own Ascension process.

CONCLUSION

If we can each take personal responsibility for raising our own consciousness, we can assist in raising the consciousness of humanity. Every one of us here on the Earth at this particular time is present for a very important reason. Each of us is a unique piece of a huge jigsaw puzzle. No two pieces are alike, and each is integral to the whole picture. By realizing this Truth, we can become more focused on our true reason for being in this embodiment. We can dedicate time through our prayers and meditation each day to fully awaken and become synchronized with our life's lessons and purpose. May you continue to be a Light in the world at this momentous time of transition on this wondrous planet Earth.

NOTES

Chapter 1

1 www.nextdimensionhealing.com.au/

2 http://in5d.com/
   how-many-of-these-51-spiritual-awakening-symptoms-do-you-have/

3 http://eftsa.com/spiritual-awakening/spiritual-awakening-using-eft/

4 Jasmuheen, *In Resonance with Jasmuheen* (Kenmore, Qld., Australia:
   Self-Empowerment Education Academy, 1998), p. 42.

5 MacDonald-Bayne, Murdo, *Spiritual and Mental Healing* (Romford,
   Essex, England: L.N. Fowler, 1947), p. 142.

6 Sutcliffe, Herbert, *How To Re-Make Your Life* (Mount Shasta, CA:
   Ascended Master Teaching Foundation, 1998), p. 79.

7 MacDonald-Bayne, *Spiritual and Mental Healing,* p. 145.

8 Sutcliffe, *How To Re-Make Your Life,* p. 48.

9 Schroeder, Werner, *The Initiations of the Seventh Ray: Compiled
   from the Teachings of the "Bridge to Freedom"* (Mount Shasta, CA:
   Ascended Master Teaching Foundation, 2008), p. 93.

10 Stone, Joshua David, and Janna Shelley Parker, *A Beginner's Guide
   to the Path of Ascension* (Sedona, AZ: Light Technology Pub., 1998),
   p. 104.

11 Sutcliffe, *How To Re-Make Your Life,* p. 78.

12 Stone and Parker, *A Beginner's Guide to the Path of Ascension,* p. 104.

13 Jasmuheen, *In Resonance with Jasmuheen* (see note 4).

14 Schroeder, Werner, *Electrons and The Elemental Kingdom: Compiled
   from the Teachings of the "Bridge to Freedom"* (Mount Shasta, CA:
   Ascended Master Teaching Foundation, 2008), p. 140.

15 Schroeder, *The Initiations of the Seventh Ray,* p. 230.

16 Jasmuheen, *In Resonance with Jasmuheen,* p. 55.

17 Besant, Annie, and C. W. Leadbeater, *Thought-forms,* Abridged ed.
   (Wheaton, IL: Theosophical Pub. House, 1969), p. 14.

18 Ibid., p. 13.

19 Ibid., p. 17.

20 Ibid., p. 29.

21 Smith, Mark, *Auras: See Them in Only 60 Seconds!* (St. Paul, MN: Llewellyn Publications, 1997), p. 5.

22 Andrews, Ted, *How to See and Read the Aura* (St. Paul, MN: Llewellyn, 1991), p. 34.

23 Ibid., p. 3.

24 Ibid.

Chapter 2

1 Schroeder, Werner, *Electrons and The Elemental Kingdom: Compiled from the Teachings of the "Bridge to Freedom"* (Mount Shasta, CA: Ascended Master Teaching Foundation, 2008), p. 218.

2 Ibid., p. 220.

3 Ibid., p. 222.

4 Jasmuheen, *In Resonance with Jasmuheen* (Kenmore, Qld., Australia: Self-Empowerment Education Academy, 1998), p. 64.

5 Leadbeater, Charles, *The Inner Life* (Wheaton, IL: Theosophical Pub., 1978), p. 153.

6 Stone, Joshua David, and Janna Shelley Parker, *A Beginner's Guide to the Path of Ascension* (Sedona, AZ: Light Technology Pub., 1998), pp. 6–13.

7 www.nextdimensionhealing.com.au/lightbodysymptoms.php

8 Hawkins, David R., *Power vs. Force: The Hidden Determinants of Human Behavior,* rev. ed. (Carlsbad, CA: Hay House, 2002), pp. 68–69.

9 Andrews, Ted, *How to See and Read the Aura* (St. Paul, MN: Llewellyn, 1991).

10 www.wangacupuncture.com/faqs.htm#faq2

11 http://umm.edu/health/medical/altmed/herb/peppermint

12 http://mentalhealthdaily.com/2014/02/25 /aromatherapy-9-best-essential-oils-for-anxiety-and-stress/

13 Goldman, Jonathan, and Andi Goldman, *Chakra Frequencies: Tantra of Sound* (Rochester, VT: Destiny Books, 2005), pp. 24–25.

Chapter 3

1 http://online.wsj.com/articles
/sleep-experts-close-in-on-the-optimal-nights-sleep-1405984970

2 http://articles.mercola.com/sites/articles/archive/2010/10/02
/secrets-to-a-good-night-sleep.aspx

3 Stone, Joshua David, *Soul Psychology: How to Clear Negative Emotions and Spiritualize Your Life* (New York: Ballantine Wellspring, Ballantine Pub. Group, 1999), p. 285.

4 Sagan, Samuel, *Entity Possession: Freeing the Energy Body of Negative Influences* (Rochester, VT: Destiny Books, 1997), p. 40.

5 Ibid.

6 Baldwin, William J., *Healing Lost Souls: Releasing Unwanted Spirits from Your Energy Body* (Charlottesville, VA: Hampton Roads Pub., 2003), p. 56.

8 Cherry, Joanna, *Self Initiations: A Manual for Spiritual Breakthrough* (Seattle, WA: Little White Buffalo Pub., 1999), p. 195.

9 Baldwin, William J., *Spirit Releasement Therapy: A Technique Manual* (Terra Alta, WV: Headline Books, 1992), p. 385.

10 Jones, Aurelia Louise, *The Seven Sacred Prayers* (Mount Shasta, CA: Mount Shasta Light Pub., 2007), p. 40.

11 MacDonald-Bayne, Murdo, *Spiritual and Mental Healing* (Romford, Essex, England: L.N. Fowler, 1947), p. 151.

12 Baldwin, *Healing Lost Souls,* pp. 257–258.

13 Kaplan, Miriam, *Crystal: The Sacred Stone* (Fallsburg, NY: Crystal Heart Press, 1988), p. 69.

14 Stone, Joshua David, and Janna Shelley Parker, *A Beginner's Guide to the Path of Ascension* (Sedona, AZ: Light Technology Pub., 1998), p. 41.

15 www.heatherruth.ws/crpkeithsmith

16 www.KeithSmithHerbShop.com

17 Schroeder, Werner, *The Angelic Kingdom: Compiled from the Teachings of the "Bridge to Freedom"* (Mount Shasta, CA: Ascended Master Teaching Foundation, 2008), p. 250.

Chapter 4

1 Papastavro, Tellis S., *The Gnosis and the Law* (Tucson, AZ: Papastavro, 1972), p. 2.

Chapter 5

1 Stone, Joshua David, *Soul Psychology: How to Clear Negative Emotions and Spiritualize Your Life* (New York: Ballantine Wellspring, Ballantine Pub. Group, 1999), p. 280.

2 Burney, Diana, *Spiritual Clearings* (Berkeley, CA: North Atlantic Books, 2009).

3 Stone, Joshua David, *Beyond Ascension: How to Complete the Seven Levels of Initiation* (Sedona, AZ: Light Technology Pub., 1995), p. 99.

4 Printz, Thomas, *The Seven Mighty Elohim Speak on the Seven Steps to Precipitation* (Mount Shasta, CA: Ascended Master Teaching Foundation, 1986), p. 28.

5 Luk, A.D.K., *The Law of Life: Book I* (Pueblo, CO: A.D.K. Luk Publications, 1989), p. 32.

6 Prophet, Elizabeth Clare, *Access the Power of Your Higher Self* (Corwin Springs, MT: Summit University Press, 1997), p. 48.

7 Luk, *The Law of Life: Book I,* p. 37.

8 Prophet, Mark L., and Elizabeth Clare Prophet, *The Science of the Spoken Word* (Livingston, MT: Summit University Press, 1991), p. 36.

9 Luk, *The Law of Life: Book I,* p. 37.

10 Baldwin, William J., *Healing Lost Souls: Releasing Unwanted Spirits from Your Energy Body* (Charlottesville, VA: Hampton Roads Pub., 2003), p. 273.

11 Baldwin, William J., *Spirit Releasement Therapy: A Technique Manual* (Terra Alta, WV: Headline Books, 1992), p. 385.

12 Luk, *The Law of Life: Book I,* p. 37.

Chapter 6

1 Luk, A.D.K. *The Law of Life: Book II* (Pueblo, CO: A.D.K. Luk Publications, 1989), pp. 254–267.

2   Printz, Thomas, *The Seven Mighty Elohim Speak on the Seven Steps to Precipitation* (Mount Shasta, CA: Ascended Master Teaching Foundation, 1986), p. 29.

3   Luk, *The Law of Life: Book II*, p. 392.

4   Ibid.

5   Luk, A.D.K., *The Law of Life: Book I* (Pueblo, CO: A.D.K. Luk Publications, 1989), p. 39.

6   Stubbs, Tony, *An Ascension Handbook: Material Channeled from Serapis* (Lithia Springs, GA: New Leaf Distributing, 1999), p. 124.

7   Cota-Robles, Patricia Diane, *The Next Step* (Tucson, AZ: New Age Study of Humanity's Purpose, Inc., 1989), p. 217.

8   Luk, *The Law of Life: Book I*, pp. 40–41.

9   Luk, *The Law of Life: Book II*, p. 393.

10 Prophet, Elizabeth Clare, *I Am Your Guard: How Archangel Michael Can Protect You* (Gardiner, MT: Summit University Press, 2008), p. 96.

11 Schroeder, Werner, *The Initiations of the Seventh Ray: Compiled from the Teachings of the "Bridge to Freedom"* (Mount Shasta, CA: Ascended Master Teaching Foundation, 2008), p. 91.

12 Stubbs, *An Ascension Handbook: Material Channeled from Serapis*, p. 124.

13 Printz, *The Seven Mighty Elohim Speak on the Seven Steps to Precipitation*, p. 225 (see note 2).

14 Schroeder, Werner, *The Angelic Kingdom: Compiled from the Teachings of the "Bridge to Freedom"* (Mount Shasta, CA: Ascended Master Teaching Foundation, 2008), p. 333.

15 Ibid., p. 351.

16 Printz, *The Seven Mighty Elohim Speak on the Seven Steps to Precipitation*, p. 225.

17 Schroeder, *The Angelic Kingdom*, p. 339.

18 Schroeder, *The Initiations of the Seventh Ray*, p. 91.

19 Luk, *The Law of Life: Book I*, p. 42.

20 Schroeder, *The Angelic Kingdom*, p. 333.

21 Printz, *The Seven Mighty Elohim Speak on the Seven Steps to Precipitation*, p. 225.

22 Luk, *The Law of Life: Book I*, p. 42.

23 Schroeder, *The Angelic Kingdom*, p. 351.

24 Cooper, Diana, *A New Light on Ascension* (Chicago: Findhorn Press, 2004), p. 26.

25 Schroeder, *The Angelic Kingdom*, p. 257.

26 Printz, *The Seven Mighty Elohim Speak on the Seven Steps to Precipitation*, pp. 191–192.

27 Luk, *The Law of Life: Book I*, p. 198.

28 Schroeder, *The Angelic Kingdom*, p. 334.

29 Schroeder, *The Initiations of the Seventh Ray*, p. 104.

30 Prophet, *I Am Your Guard: How Archangel Michael Can Protect You*, p. 98 (see note 10).

31 Ibid., p. 99.

32 Schroeder, *The Initiations of the Seventh Ray*, p. 145.

33 Ibid.

34 Cooper, *A New Light on Ascension*, p. 27 (see note 24).

35 Prophet, Mark, and Elizabeth Clare Prophet, *The Science of the Spoken Word* (Livingston, MT: Summit University Press, 1983), p. 113.

36 Prophet, Elizabeth Clare, and Patricia R. Spadaro, *Alchemy of the Heart: How to Give and Receive More Love* (Corwin Springs, MT: Summit University Press, 2000), p. 128.

37 Prophet and Prophet, *The Science of the Spoken Word*, p. 116.

38 Printz, *The Seven Mighty Elohim Speak on the Seven Steps to Precipitation*, p. 225.

39 Ibid.

40 Cota-Robles, Patricia Diane, *Your Time Is At Hand* (Tucson, AZ: New Age Study of Humanity's Purpose, 1992), p. 98.

41 Cameron, Pam, and Fred Cameron, *Bridge into Light*, 2nd ed. (Livermore, CA: Oughten House, 1994), p. 97.

42 Schroeder, *The Initiations of the Seventh Ray*, p. 145.

43 Printz, *The Seven Mighty Elohim Speak on the Seven Steps to Precipitation,* p. 225.

44 Schroeder, *The Angelic Kingdom,* p. 334.

Chapter 7

1 Jasmuheen, *In Resonance with Jasmuheen* (Kenmore, Qld., Australia: Self-Empowerment Education Academy, 1998), p. 23.

2 Luk, A.D.K., *The Law of Life: Book II* (Pueblo, CO: A.D.K. Luk Publications, 1989), p. 401.

3 Papastavro, Tellis S., *The Gnosis and the Law* (Tucson, AZ: Papastavro, 1972), p. 216.

4 Schroeder, Werner, *Electrons and The Elemental Kingdom: Compiled from the Teachings of the "Bridge to Freedom"* (Mount Shasta, CA: Ascended Master Teaching Foundation, 2008), p. 130.

5 Luk, *The Law of Life: Book II,* p. 400.

6 Luk, A.D.K., *The Law of Life: Book I* (Pueblo, CO: A.D.K. Luk Publications, 1989), p. 37.

7 Jones, Aurelia Louise, *The Seven Sacred Flames* (Mount Shasta, CA: Mount Shasta Light Pub., 2007), p. 15.

8 Luk, *The Law of Life: Book II,* p. 400.

9 Ibid., p. 437.

10 Ibid., p. 401.

11 Ibid.

12 Ibid.

13 Ibid., pp. 294–95.

14 Stone, Joshua David, and Janna Shelley Parker, *A Beginner's Guide to the Path of Ascension* (Sedona, AZ: Light Technology Pub., 1998), p. 105.

15 http//.dymamoh.com.au

16 Stone and Parker, *A Beginner's Guide to the Path of Ascension,* p. 105.

17 Crowley, Brian, and Esther Crowley, *Words of Power: Sacred Sounds of East & West* (St. Paul, MN: Llewellyn Publications, 1991), p. 161.

18 Stone and Parker, *A Beginner's Guide to the Path of Ascension,* p. 105.

19 Prophet, Elizabeth Clare, and Patricia R. Spadaro, *Alchemy of the Heart: How to Give and Receive More Love* (Corwin Springs, MT: Summit University Press, 2000), p. 151.

20 Kuthumi and Djwal Kul, dictated to Mark L. Prophet and Elizabeth Clare Prophet, *The Human Aura: How to Activate and Energize Your Aura and Chakras* (Livingston, MT: Summit University Press, 1996), p. 371.

21 Schroeder, Werner, *The Initiations of the Seventh Ray: Compiled from the Teachings of the "Bridge to Freedom"* (Mount Shasta, CA: Ascended Master Teaching Foundation, 2008), p. 228.

22 Luk, *The Law of Life: Book I,* p. 170.

23 Ibid., p. 172.

24 Prophet, Elizabeth Clare, *I Am Your Guard: How Archangel Michael Can Protect You* (Gardiner, MT: Summit University Press, 2008), pp. 100–101.

25 Ibid., pp. 78–79.

26 Stone, Joshua David, *Soul Psychology: How to Clear Negative Emotions and Spiritualize Your Life* (New York: Ballantine Wellspring, Ballantine Pub. Group, 1999), p. 295.

27 Scheffer, Mechthild, *Bach Flower Therapy: Theory and Practice* (Rochester, VT: Healing Arts Press, 1988), p. 16.

28 Jones, Anne, *Healing Negative Energies* (London: Piatkus, 2002), pp. 74–75.

29 *Essential Oils Desk Reference,* 5th ed. (Lehi, UT: Life Science Pub., 2011), p. 12.

30 Ibid., p. 12.

31 Jones, *Healing Negative Energies,* p. 74.

32 http://hawaiianwellness.com/about2/

33 www.crossroad.to/Books/sumbols/htm.

34 Griscom, Chris, *The Healing of Emotion: Awakening the Fearless Self* (New York: Simon and Schuster, 1990).

35 teacherpress.ocps.net/patriciadavis/files/.../Macromolecule-Worksheet

36 Cameron, Pam, and Fred Cameron, *Bridge into Light,* 2nd ed. (Livermore, CA: Oughten House, 1994), pp. 1–5.

37 Ibid., pp. 1–6.

38 Ibid.

39 This information from multiple sources is too large to list.

40 Stone and Parker, *A Beginner's Guide to the Path of Ascension,* p. 107 (see note 14).

41 Ibid.

42 Mitchell, Wayne, *New Heart English Bible* (Bloomington, IN: AuthorHouse, 2008), Matthew 6:9–13.

43 Bailey, Alice, *The Seven Rays of Life* (New York: Lucis Pub., 1995).

44 www.lucistrust.org

45 www.unity.org/resources/articles/prayer-protection

46 Two Disciples, *The Rainbow Bridge: First Phase Link with the Soul* (Los Angeles: New Age Press, 1975).

47 www.magicofgayatri.com/pages/magic-of-gayatri.html

48 www.lucistrust.org/en/service_activities/e_mantrams/the_gayatri

49 Vanzant, Iyanla, *Everyday I Pray: Awakening to the Grace of Inner Communion* (New York: Simon and Schuster, 2002).

50 Walker, Dael, *The Crystal Healing Book* (Pacheco, CA: Crystal, 1988).

51 www.lucistrust.org/en/service_activities/e_mantrams /the_mantram_of_unification

52 Jones, Aurelia Louise, *The Seven Sacred Flames* (Mount Shasta, CA: Mount Shasta Light Pub., 2007), p. 51.

53 Stone and Parker, *A Beginner's Guide to the Path of Ascension,* p. 108.

Chapter 8

1 Barton, Ruth H., *Sacred Rhythms: Arranging Our Lives for Spiritual Transformation* (Downers Grove, IL: InterVarsity Press, 2006), p. 148.

2 Blaze, Chrissie, *Workout for the Soul: Eight Steps to Inner Fitness* (Fairfield, CT: Aslan Pub., 2001), pp. 143–49.

3 Peirce, Penney, *Frequency: The Power of Personal Vibration* (New York: Atria Books 2009), p. 47.

4 Ibid., p. 49.

5 Schroeder, Werner, *Electrons and The Elemental Kingdom: Compiled from the Teachings of the "Bridge to Freedom"* (Mount Shasta, CA: Ascended Master Teaching Foundation, 2008), p. 133.

6 Peirce, *Frequency: The Power of Personal Vibration*, p. 49.

7 Ibid., p. 118.

8 Cousens, Gabriel, *Spiritual Nutrition and the Rainbow Diet* (Boulder, CO: Cassandra Press, 1986), p. 74. This book was republished by North Atlantic Books in 2005.

9 Ibid., p. 76.

10 Cousins, David, and Jean Prince, *A Handbook for Light Workers* (Dartmouth, UK: Barton House, 1993), p. 89.

11 Ibid., p. 90.

Chapter 9

1 Ingerman, Sandra, *Soul Retrieval: Mending the Fragmented Self* (San Francisco, CA: HarperSanFrancisco, 1991), pp. 12–14.

2 Ibid., pp. 22–23.

3 Baldwin, William J., *Healing Lost Souls: Releasing Unwanted Spirits from Your Energy Body* (Charlottesville, VA: Hampton Roads Pub., 2003), pp. 46–47.

4 Source unknown

5 Ingerman, *Soul Retrieval*, pp. 104–13.

6 Baldwin, *Healing Lost Souls*, p. 273.

Chapter 10

1 Jasmuheen, *In Resonance with Jasmuheen* (Kenmore, Qld., Australia: Self-Empowerment Education Academy, 1998), p. 90.

Chapter 12

1 Hawkins, David R., *Power vs. Force: The Hidden Determinants of Human Behavior*, Rev. ed. (Carlsbad, CA: Hay House, 2002).

2 Peirce, Penney, *Frequency: The Power of Personal Vibration* (New York: Atria Books, 2009), p. 32.

3 Sagan, Samuel, *Entity Possession: Freeing the Energy Body of Negative Influences* (Rochester, VT: Destiny Books, 1997), p. 133.

4 Ibid., p. 134.

5 Wallace, Amy, and Bill Henkin, *The Psychic Healing Book* (New York: Delacorte Press, 1978), pp. 79–84.

6 Papastavro, Tellis S., *The Gnosis and the Law* (Tucson, AZ: Papastavro, 1972), p. 244.

7 Schroeder, Werner, *Electrons and The Elemental Kingdom: Compiled from the Teachings of the "Bridge to Freedom"* (Mount Shasta, CA: Ascended Master Teaching Foundation, 2008), p. 250.

8 Ibid., p. 257.

9 Luk, A.D.K., *The Law of Life: Book II* (Pueblo, CO: A.D.K. Luk Publications, 1989), p. 215.

10 Barton, Ruth H., *Sacred Rhythms: Arranging Our Lives for Spiritual Transformation* (Downers Grove, IL: InterVarsity Press, 2006), pp. 176–77.

11 Jasmuheen, *In Resonance with Jasmuheen* (Kenmore, Qld., Australia: Self-Empowerment Education Academy, 1998), p. 46.

12 www.masaru-emoto.net/english/water-crystal.html

Chapter 13

1 Printz, Thomas, *The Seven Mighty Elohim Speak on the Seven Steps to Precipitation* (Mount Shasta, CA: Ascended Master Teaching Foundation, 1986), p. 225.

2 Andrews, Ted, *How to Heal with Color* (St. Paul, MN: Llewellyn Publications, 1992), p. 110.

3 Crowley, Brian, and Esther Crowley, *Words of Power: Sacred Sounds of East & West* (St. Paul, MN: Llewellyn Publications, 1991), p. 152.

4 Ibid., p. 151.

5 MacDonald-Bayne, Murdo, *Spiritual and Mental Healing* (Romford, Essex, England: L.N. Fowler, 1947), p. 22.

6 Ibid., p. 23.

Chapter 14

1 Jasmuheen, *In Resonance with Jasmuheen* (Kenmore, Qld., Australia: Self-Empowerment Education Academy, 1998), p. 81.

2 Ibid., p. 148.

3 Ibid., p. 64.

4 Schroeder, Werner. *The Initiations of the Seventh Ray: Compiled from the Teachings of the "Bridge to Freedom"* (Mount Shasta, CA: Ascended Master Teaching Foundation, 2008), pp. 91–92.

5 MacDonald-Bayne, Murdo, *Spiritual and Mental Healing* (Romford, Essex, England: L.N. Fowler, 1947).

6 Stone, Joshua David, *Soul Psychology: How to Clear Negative Emotions and Spiritualize your Life* (New York: Ballantine Wellspring, Ballantine Pub. Group, 1999), p. 49.

7 Schroeder, Werner, *Electrons and The Elemental Kingdom: Compiled from the Teachings of the "Bridge to Freedom"* (Mount Shasta, CA: Ascended Master Teaching Foundation, 2008), pp. 293–294.

8 Ibid., p. 293.

9 Luk, A.D.K., *The Law of Life: Book II* (Pueblo, CO: A.D.K. Luk Publications, 1989), p. 399.

10 Ibid., p. 439.

11 Kuthumi and Djwal Kul, dictated to Mark L. Prophet and Elizabeth Clare Prophet, *The Human Aura: How to Activate and Energize Your Aura and Chakras* (Livingston, MT: Summit University Press, 1996), p. 423.

12 The Ascended Master Hilarion, *A Primer on Healing: Basic Knowledge and Basic Practice* (New York: The New Age Church of The Christ, 1981).

13 Leadbeater, C. W., *The Masters and the Path* (Chicago: Theosophical Press, 1925), p. 196.

14 Stone, Joshua David, *The Complete Ascension Manual: How to Achieve Ascension in This Lifetime* (Sedona, AZ: Light Technology Pub., 1994), p. 128.

15 Kuthumi and Djwal Kul, *The Human Aura,* p. 418 (see note 11).

16 Leadbeater, *The Masters and the Path,* pp. 197–204.

17 Stone, *Soul Psychology,* pp. 214–215 (see note 6).

18 Ibid.

19 Ibid.

20 Ibid.

21 Ibid.

22 Ibid.

23 Ibid.

24 Jones, Aurelia Louise, *The Seven Sacred Flames* (Mount Shasta, CA: Mount Shasta Light Pub., 2007), p. 58.

Chapter 15

1 Source unknown.

2 VOICE of the "I AM," July 1945.

3 Lin, Chunyi, *Spring Forest Qigong: Level I for Health* (United States: Chunyi Lin, 2000).

4 Ibid.

Chapter 16

1 Jones, Aurelia Louise, *Prayers to the Seven Sacred Flames* (Mount Shasta, CA: Mount Shasta Light Pub., 2007), p. 55.

2 Cota-Robles, Patricia Diane, *The Next Step* (Tucson, AZ: New Age Study of Humanity's Purpose, Inc., 1989), p. 234.

3 Ibid.

4 Ibid., p. 235.

5 Cherry, Joanna, *Self Initiations: A Manual for Spiritual Breakthrough* (Seattle, WA: Little White Buffalo Pub., 1999), p. 192.

6 Jones, Aurelia Louise, *The Seven Sacred Flames,* (Mount Shasta, CA: Mount Shasta Light Pub., 2007), p. 58.

7 Schroeder, Werner, *Electrons and The Elemental Kingdom: Compiled from the Teachings of the "Bridge to Freedom"* (Mount Shasta, CA: Ascended Master Teaching Foundation, 2008).

8 Ibid., p. 204.

9 Ibid., pp. 302–303.

10 Ibid., p. 264.

11 Ibid., pp. 304–305.

12 Ibid., p. 264.

13 Ibid., pp. 306–307.

14 Ibid., p. 263.

15 Ibid., pp. 308–309.

INDEX

ACKNOWLEDGMENTS

It is with deep gratitude that I thank the following for assisting me with the creation of this book: All my Guides and Teachers of 100% pure Light, and the Ascended Masters and the Archangels for their love, guidance, and inspiration.

Special gratitude to Richard Grossinger of North Atlantic Books for his acceptance of my manuscript and also his assistance and intention as a publisher to provide spiritually focused books to readers; Tim McKee and the Acquisition Committee for choosing this manuscript and having faith in the project; Marcia Schmidt for her support and for introducing me to Richard; Vanessa Ta, Project Editor, for keeping me on task with deadlines and for all her suggestions and assistance; and my copy editor, Kathy Glass, for her assistance in the book's final form.

I would also like to express sincere thanks to the following for their contributions in developing this book: Tana Dean for the formatting of the manuscript; Sanaya Roman for her suggestions and support; Suzie Kiefer, Susan Major, and Sister Mary Dean and the Lial Renewal Center for providing the conditions I needed to write this book; Christine Taft, Susan O'Connor, Francesca Militeau, and Paula Snelling for their enthusiasm, contributions, and valuable feedback; Marshall Govindan, my Kriya Yoga Teacher, for bestowing upon me my spiritual name of Savitri; and much gratitude also to the people who have reviewed and/ or endorsed the book, including Nora Caron, Elise and Kaleo Ching, LaUna Huffines, Dr. Robert Alcorn, and Amara Mahduri. I also must acknowledge my Higher Self for facilitating a large portion of this text through my automatic writing process.

My heartfelt thanks and gratitude also go to the following individuals: my sister Kristy for her unconditional love and her encouragement and support all along the way; my daughters Kimberly and Kelley, and my grandchildren Avery and Quinn, who have all given me the opportunity to love fully. I also wish to acknowledge the following: all past, present, and future students and clients; those who have assisted me on my spiritual journey, both known and unknown; and all who read this book and use the information to improve the quality of their life on their spiritual path.

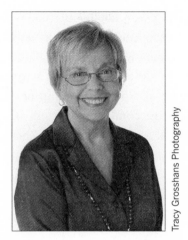

Tracy Grosshans Photography

ABOUT THE AUTHOR

DIANA BURNEY, RN, BSN, MEd, has more than forty years' experience in management, counseling, marketing, and education. She developed successful private counseling practices in four states, while remaining current with appropriate credentials for the health care arena. She is a registered nurse, certified hypnotherapist, and ordained minister of the Order of Melchizedek from the Sanctuary of the Beloved in Conesus, New York. She is also a certified Reiki Master/Teacher as well as a Magnified Healing Practitioner. She holds a master's in education from Cleveland State University and a Doctorate of Divinity degree from The College of Divine Metaphysics in Glendora, California. Burney has done thousands of Clearings for properties, individuals, and animals for nearly twenty-five years. These Clearings have been done in every state in the U.S. and more than eighty foreign countries. She has been featured in *SPA* magazine; and articles have been written in the *Toronto Star* and *Florida-Times Union* about her success with remote Energy Clearings for homes and property.

Burney has appeared on various cable TV and radio shows including *Coast to Coast* with Art Bell and *The Uri Geller Show.* She has been teaching Spiritual Clearing Weekend Intensives for more than fifteen years. She has written the following online articles: "The Importance of Discernment," "Developing the Intuitive Mind," and "Breaking Free from the Past." In 2013 she was an anchor writer for an international online publication with a strong readership of 24,000 women worldwide (www.sibylmagazine.com). In addition, Burney is the author of the award-winning book *Spiritual Clearings*. She currently lives in Ann Arbor, Michigan, and has been the president of Earth Release since 1999 and founder of Healing Vibrations since 2001. She is available for speaking engagements, interviews, and appearances. Burney can be reached through her Earth Release website: www.earthrelease.com.

Praise for *Spiritual Balancing*

"*Spiritual Balancing* is a valuable compilation of virtually unknown spiritual teachers. [Burney] writes for beginners on a spiritual path and includes practical suggestions and practices from her own spiritual journey."

—LaUna Huffines, author of *Healing Yourself with Light*

"At a time when our world is threatened by adverse effects of human endeavor, *Spiritual Balancing* offers hope and wise guidance for reclaiming our collective journey toward the highest good for ourselves, the earth, and all who dwell here with us."

—Elise and Kaleo Ching, authors of *The Creative Art of Living, Dying, and Renewal*

"Diana's latest self-help book, *Spiritual Balancing,* is packed with relevant spiritual tools and tips for dealing with the new energies hitting Earth. I found myself learning so much new information that my head was spinning with all the possibilities ahead!"

—Nora Caron, author of *Journey to the Heart, New Dimensions of Being,* and *Jaguar Dreams*

"Diana has put together a concise and illuminated compendium of wisdom for today's seekers."

—Patricia Cori, author of the *Sirian Revelations* trilogy